HuD

Please renew or return items by the date shown on your receipt

www.hertsdirect.org/libraries

Renewals and enquiries: 0300 123 4049

Textphone for hearing or speech impaired 0300 123 4041

Hertfordshire

D1350643

467 765 31 X

The *Blissful* Baby Expert

Everything you need to know
for easier, happier parenting

LISA CLEGG

Vermilion
LONDON

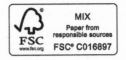

To Jack, Ollie & Loren – my own three amazing 'blissful babies'.

Contents

Foreword

Bringing a baby home for the first time must be one of the most daunting experiences anyone can face. Suddenly there is very small, odd, cute little person who is relying on you to keep her alive. And if, at any point, you neglect one of her very, very many needs and wants, you know about it in the most certain terms.

I was under no illusions that I could wing it when I had my first daughter. I'd never been around small babies, had no idea how they operated and had no desire to rely on something as unpredictable as 'instinct'. I booked Lisa to help me through those first few hellish weeks, and I would say that not only did she teach me to be a proper, instinctive mother, she allowed me to enjoy my tiny baby more than I ever thought possible.

Her methods felt natural, in tune with my baby's natural rhythm rather than trying to impose a stringent routine on a capricious little baby. Occasionally, I would get told by elderly relatives that I should 'let my baby find its own routine'. Yet, my baby seemed so happy on Lisa's sleeping and eating plan while those left to 'find their own routine' seemed to cry all the time.

As a nervous, novice mother, I found it immensely reassuring that I knew roughly when my baby would sleep or eat. It meant that if she was crying, I could immediately rule out at least one or two causes. I'd seen so many of my friends fall into the trap of feeding a crying baby whose real problem was wind, causing their baby real pain.

I was also, though it is difficult to confess in these highly charged times, a reluctant breastfeeder. I wasn't at all sure about the idea at first, even though I knew it would be great for my baby. I fully planned to give up after a couple of weeks. Lisa's methods made it so easy that I ended up breastfeeding for around six months with both my babies.

Ultimately, so many people said I was 'lucky' that I had two babies that fed and slept so well. I put this all down to Lisa's methods. My second daughter is completely wild, a total tearaway, yet she has always slept well, which has made it so much easier to cope with her energetic nature. It is the only predictable thing about her.

I am so glad that other people will now have the opportunity to use Lisa's methods and have happy little babies of their own. It will never quite beat having her in person, but I was very lucky. There is a lifetime's worth of experience of little babies in this book. At its heart is a desire to have a happy baby and a happy mother. My 'babies' are now two and four and the sleep patterns they learned in those early days have, I believe, set them up perfectly for life.

Cherry Reynard, mother to Hannah and Lexi

About the author

I grew up the fourth eldest of 26 grandchildren, so I have been surrounded by babies and small children from a young age. I've always been particularly interested in small babies and I was always the one who volunteered to take any babies off their parents' hands at family get-togethers and parties!

All I ever wanted to do when I left school was to get a job working with children. Many schoolteachers tried to discourage me from going into the childcare sector, reasoning that I was wasting my good exam results wanting to go into a job involving children, which tended to be very poorly paid. I was very determined though, and after leaving school I went straight to college to do the NNEB-Diploma in Childcare and Education, which is equivalent to an NVQ Level 3 in childcare. The NNEB is now known as the CACHE Diploma.

After completing the two-year course I went straight into my first nanny position, where I had sole charge of three children aged six, four and six months. Another baby was born within the two years that I spent working for the family. I loved my time with them and the job made me realise that I definitely wanted to continue nannying, as I enjoyed the personal relationship you are able to build with both the children and their parents.

Feeling prepared for motherhood I continued in nannying up until I had my first baby, Jack, in October 2002.

After a short spell of maternity leave, I was lucky enough to be able to take my baby to work with me and care for him alongside the children. Jack was a very easy baby who happily ate and slept wherever he was. But having my baby in a good routine was even more essential for me because of work. He was breastfed from the start but also offered one bottle of expressed milk per day from the age of two weeks, which meant my husband could get involved with feeding him, and allow me to catch up on some much-needed sleep! Jack continued to be a very happy baby and slotted into my work routine easily.

When he was three years old I began to work two days per week in a nursery and he enjoyed some social time mixing with other children. I worked in the baby room with children up to two years but my care was mainly for babies aged from birth to 12 months. I had always resisted working in nurseries before as I loved the freedom that nannying gave me, but the job offer helped our personal childcare situation at the time, and I surprised myself by loving working with the babies even in a nursery environment.

After my second son was born in 2006, I began doing some maternity night-nanny contracts. I discovered night nannying by accident as I browsed through a childcare job website. Like many people, I knew that some mothers employ someone to come and live in and help them after the birth of their baby. However, I didn't realise that a mother could employ someone just to do the nights, allowing her the crucial part of the day covered so that she could get some sleep. Having just gone through the sleepless nights myself with my second baby, I knew first-hand how torturous it can be when feel like you will never get a full night's sleep again. A good night's sleep means you feel like you can cope with anything during the day!

I absolutely loved the night nannying as it gave me access to the age group I loved working with the most – those tiny newborns – and I knew exactly how the mothers I worked for would be feeling. It wasn't long before I realised that this was the job I wanted to do long term. It meant being self-employed and not having guaranteed work, which was precarious for the family finances but I can honestly say it was the best decision I could have made. I have been busy since that day. I love my job and get so much satisfaction from starting work with a new family, who are usually in chaos with neither parent knowing quite where to start. It's fantastic to leave happy parents that are confident about caring for their happy baby, who eats and sleeps well!

Introduction

When my children are crying it upsets me too. When they are hurt I want to be able to take away the pain. When they are ill I would happily take their place so that they are well again. This is a completely natural parental reaction, and as parents all any of us want for our children is to see them happy.

To see their smiling faces enjoying something they are doing or laughing at something they have seen is what makes all the hard parts of being a parent worthwhile!

As a mother of three children, I know how important this is in everyday life. Happy babies and children equal happy parents, so it's only right that we as parents try to do our best to enable our babies to develop into happy children from the day they are born!

There are so many baby books on the market telling parents the right and the wrong things they should or shouldn't do with their baby, and it's so difficult knowing which method to use, particularly when they all seem to contradict each other. 'Feed your baby on demand', 'let them find their own routine', are common phrases in books and from our local health visitors and midwives. They are trained to promote NHS and UNICEF guidelines, but it is worth remembering these are precisely that: 'guidelines'. When it comes to raising children, there is no one-size-fits-all as every baby is unique. Mothers are often made to feel like they are doing something wrong, or being unfair to their baby, by wanting some sort of daily routine to give both their baby and themselves some sort of stability and structure on a regular basis.

There are also books on the market that are very strict with routine – both for the babies *and* the mothers – with barely any room for flexibility. In families where there is more than one child this just doesn't work. With school runs to fit in and mothers having to return to work, routines have to be adapted to suit everyone's needs at times. Life does have to go on and can't always be focused on sticking 100 per cent to the baby's routine.

However, this book has been written to give mothers a daily guideline to follow to make life a lot easier and happier for everyone from day one. All babies are different though and will need slightly different amounts of sleep: some need 15–30 minutes more than others at the various sleep times. Therefore it will be down to the parent to gauge exactly what works for their individual baby, based on the routine provided. I would never be able to give you a routine that will work exactly for every single baby, and anyone who says that is possible is being unrealistic. Babies are not robots and all have completely different personalities, so each routine needs to be tweaked slightly and adapted in terms of the amount of sleep needed to suit each particular baby.

In using this routine as a basis and gently steering babies in the right direction from day one, at the end of each contract I have left happy parents whose babies typically drop their night feed between eight and ten weeks, settle well during sleep times and are in general very relaxed, happy babies. It won't happen overnight but with lots of patience and perseverance – what I like to call the two Ps – you too can have a happy baby who eats, sleeps and plays very contentedly and actually doesn't need to cry, as their needs are always met!

It has worked for many mums and babies, and it was all of them that inspired me to write this book. I wanted to reach out to so many more parents who are desperate for answers to basic questions and who just need someone to point them in the right direction to keep life with a newborn baby on an even keel. This book is here to give you that starting block, and as a mother of three children myself I understand first-hand how difficult life with a newborn can be when you are not sure where to begin.

Is a routine for you?

Establishing a routine can help you feel more in control of what is happening on a day-to-day basis and keep sleep deprivation to a minimum rather than becoming overwhelmed by it! A routine gives the main carer and the baby a daily structure, which makes life a lot easier and happier for everyone in the long run. The baby will be happier because she never gets a chance to become overtired and irritable, she will be fed regularly during the day and will be getting the correct amount of stimulation. The parent, in turn, is happier because having a routine means other things can be planned to fit in around feed and sleep times.

Achieving small things like having a shower or hanging some washing out, without feeling totally stressed, is not easy if your baby is not in a routine. Most babies generally find their own routine eventually, but much later on, when they are older. To get to that stage without any routine would have likely been a long haul of more sleep-deprived nights and fractious days than are necessary. Babies simply don't need to be so unhappy. The ability to sleep properly is a gift for life and needs to be taught.

Guilt

Many parents refrain from attempting a routine from an early age because of the guilt attached. Guilt comes not just from other people but also from within ourselves. Let's face it: you will always have feelings of guilt. Guilt is all part and parcel of becoming a mother. It starts from the day your baby is born, and you feel guilty about everything you do or don't do from that day onwards. It is a perfectly normal everyday feeling, particularly for mothers. Generally speaking, guilt doesn't seem to be something that blights fathers. Of course, they love and care for their babies as much as mothers do, and equally would lay down their own life to protect their child. However, in my experience men seem to be able to 'switch off' that worry that constantly plagues us mothers every minute of the day, whether we are with our babies or apart from them for any length of time.

In talking to many mothers with babies and children of varying ages, I don't think the guilt ever goes away. I still feel terribly guilty when I send my 11-year-old son to his room and take away his privileges as a punishment for something he's done, even though I know I have to do it for his own benefit – and my own sanity!

It would be very easy for us all to give in to our babies and children's wants every step of the way. It may make them happy initially in the short term, but in the long run you will be doing their social development no favours at all. In doing this they will begin to expect everything their own way constantly, and be more likely to have behavioural problems when you are at home and out and about. I've never wanted to be one of those mothers whose child is kicking and screaming in the middle of the cereal aisle at the supermarket while everyone walking past looks on in pity.

> **Tip**
> *What you need to remember is that there is a big difference between meeting your baby's needs and just giving in to her demands and wants!*

Although we know in our heads that certain stages our babies go through are normal and part and parcel of them growing up, it doesn't make you feel any less guilty about them. Dropping the night feed, moving her from a basket to the big cot, stopping breastfeeding, moving from a bottle to a cup, leaving her to cry for any length of time. These are all phases that will generate huge feelings of guilt by just considering implementing them, let alone actually doing them!

I find that it helps knowing these feelings are normal and that you are in the same boat as everyone else. Guilt will never be something you can control. It's more something that you learn to live with as you make the changes necessary for your and your baby's well-being. Think of it as nature's way of making sure you look after your baby properly.

Friends and family members can be very judgemental at times about how you bring up your baby. The crucial thing that you need to remember and keep reminding yourself of is that it is *your* baby, and as a parent you can only ever do what you think is best for all of you.

Motherhood is not a battle against other mothers – it is *your* journey with *your* child or children.

It doesn't matter what anyone else thinks. As long as you, your baby and the rest of the family living in your house are happy then that's all that matters.

There is no way to be a perfect mother, but there are a million ways to be a good one, and that's all we can strive to be!

Remember: happy babies equal happy parents! Good luck!

For the purposes of this book, and to save constantly writing he/she or mother/father, I have written with my youngest child in mind, a girl, Loren, and me, 'Mum', the main carer.

1

Before your baby is born

The baby equipment market worldwide is worth millions. With so many different brands to choose from, it can be very daunting knowing what essential items to buy, what are 'nice' to have around and those things that will never be used! It's very important to get all the equipment you will need to last you the first three months before the birth. Larger items like highchairs, baby walkers and weaning items can all be purchased after the birth when your baby is old enough to need them. I have listed items under the headings of 'essential', 'helpful' and 'not needed' and then explained my reasons. Family members or friends may offer to buy various items for you, so you can use the list below to give them an option of what to buy.

Getting ready
- Your hospital bag should be packed and ready from around 32 weeks of pregnancy. It is always best to be well prepared just in case you go into premature labour. It would add more stress to an already pressured situation if you had to rely on a partner or family member to try to find and pack all of the items you and the baby needed because you hadn't got your hospital bag pre-packed in an emergency situation. See Chapter 2 for recommended items to pack.
- If there are any important birthdays coming up in the month after your due date that you don't want to forget, then it's a

good idea to buy cards and presents in advance. This will save time and effort later, and relieve the pressure on you when you would rather be focusing on your new baby.

- If you can, try to cook some meals and freeze them in advance before the birth. This will make the weeks after your baby is born easier, as you can just defrost a healthy home-cooked meal and pop it into the oven or microwave to heat up, rather than trying to find time to cook something from scratch. Casseroles, shepherd's pie, lasagne, stir-fry and curries are all examples of meals that can be frozen into portions. It will be important to eat regularly and healthily after the birth to help your body recover. It is even more important when breastfeeding as what you eat will also be feeding your baby.

Equipment to buy

The items and equipment I have included in this chapter are the things I found most useful when my babies were born and also things that other parents have recommended to me. There may be other items you feel are essential to your family when your baby is born, to compliment your lifestyle and environment, which you can add to the list. I just wanted to give you a starting block of where to begin, as I remember how daunting the world of baby equipment was when pregnant with my first child!

The basics

Cot (essential)

There are so many colours, makes and shapes of cot on the market. Where do you start? Cot or cot bed? To be honest there isn't a right or wrong one to buy – it will usually come down to the colour you prefer and whether it matches the nursery. The size will depend on the size of your baby's room. As long as your final choice meets all of the current safety regulations then it will be absolutely fine whether it costs £50 or £500! The current British

Standard safety standard that all baby cots have to adhere to is the BS1753.

It is sometimes easier to buy a **cot bed** rather than just a cot purely because it will last longer, although these are bigger than a standard cot so that may be a factor in your choice. Cot beds are more expensive to buy, but once your baby is a toddler you will be able to take the sides off and it will turn into a bed, which can last until your child is around five years old.

Most cots now come with **teething rails** along the top bars. These are clear plastic covers that go over the wood. Once your little one can pull herself to standing, the height of the top bar is just perfect for her to gnaw on. Trust me, they love to do it – as all three of my children did! Having the teething rail makes it a little more hygienic for babies to chew on rather than them just biting the bare wood, as you can give it a wipe regularly. It's worth choosing a cot that already has these, although they can be purchased separately.

It's very important to buy a good quality ventilated **mattress** for the cot that meets the current British safety standard BS1877 and BS7177. I recommend buying a new one for each baby you have and not reusing a sibling's mattress or buying a second-hand one. Remember this is somewhere your baby will sleep every night for 12–13 hours as well as daytime naps for the next two to three years, even longer in the case of cot bed mattresses. She will sweat on hot days and certainly vomit on it at some point. Even though it will be covered with a cot sheet, the sweat and vomit stains can still go through on to the mattress. At least if it's a new mattress the germs are all from your baby only, which is much safer and more hygienic! In some cases you may find that the mattress will actually cost you more than the cot itself, but it is definitely worth making sure you get the right one. If you go to a big baby superstore they will advise you and recommend the correct mattress for the cot you plan to buy.

Moses basket (helpful and practical)

This is not a completely essential item. If you prefer, the baby can sleep in a big cot from the day she comes home from hospital. You can either put her in a cot in the nursery on the first night home and thereafter, or set the cot up in your room for the first few weeks to make things easier for night feeds. It can then be moved to the nursery once your baby drops her night feed.

However, in my opinion a Moses basket can be a very practical item to have in the first 10 weeks or so. Ninety-five per cent of the parents I have worked for used one – by their own choice, not my recommendation – which they've often borrowed from a relative. I used one for my three children and all of my friends and family did too, all for the same reason.

When you have just had a baby you don't want her in another room at night-time. As a parent you want to keep an eye on your children and make sure they are okay and safe at all times – show me the parent that doesn't spend those early days checking the rise and fall of their little one's chest! Half the time you won't even realise you are doing it! I used to wake myself up as I had been dreaming the baby had been crying, which is what many parents do. Generally you find that the baby is still fast asleep, and you are just hearing things as you are on high alert in preparation for your baby's cries! It's much easier to check her if she is next to you. Therefore, most parents would not be happy to put their newborn in a completely different room to them in those early days or weeks.

Sadly a cot takes up a fair amount of room and wouldn't fit in most parents' bedrooms without using up precious space, so a Moses basket is the next best option. It's small and portable so can move from room to room, or even downstairs if needed.

In the first few weeks babies do not mind or even notice which room they sleep in as long as their sleep environment and routine remains the same – i.e., same cot/Moses basket, so their comforting smells remain the same. They wouldn't mind if the basket were put in another room on any given night. This may need to happen if a kindly grandparent or friend were to offer some much-needed relief for you at night-time. You can then easily move the basket into a spare room. The same couldn't be said for a cot.

Once the baby is older and no longer needs to be fed in the night, and perhaps has grown too big for the Moses basket, she can be moved to the big cot in the nursery for her sleeps. By this time you are usually emotionally ready for this to happen anyway, as she is not so small any more.

I have never had any babies who have problems settling or sleeping when we do the transition from Moses basket to cot as it's usually done in the first 8–12 weeks depending on the parents' choice and the babies' size. You can get your baby used to her cot and nursery environment by putting her in the cot during the day. Some parents find a good time to do this is when you are getting her bath ready. You could put her mobile on for her to watch while you sort everything out ready to bathe her.

Cot mobile (helpful)

I think a cot mobile is a really good thing to have, and it's a really fun thing to choose too. It can be used as a sleep prompt and indicator to your baby that it is time to go to sleep. You don't need to spend a fortune on one with all sorts of lullabies and lights that make pretty patterns on the wall; in fact I would positively discourage any kind of mobile that creates any sort of light show, as this will just act as a stimulant to your baby. In my opinion the best mobiles to buy are the basic wind-up ones with three or four animals hanging down. This will spin round as a tune plays when you wind it up before leaving the baby's room, and she will very quickly learn this as a cue to go to sleep. Try to choose one in a strong colour. White or cream mobiles look very neat but your new baby's vision will take a few weeks to improve, so she will enjoy a brightly coloured mobile a lot more.

Pushchair/pram (essential)

Obviously this is an essential item. Choices such as style and colour are individual to each parent. As long as it complies with the safety standard, there is no right or wrong one to buy. You do need to make sure that it lies completely flat for your newborn though and has a five-point harness in the case of a pushchair. Other helpful things to look for are:

- Is there a rain cover included?
- Does it have a shopping basket?
- Does it fold easily with one hand? This is essential if you will be using buses regularly, as you will have a baby in the other arm!
- Does it have a built-in hood/sun shade?
- Does it have a brake?
- Does it have swivel wheels? These make pushing and turning corners much easier!
- Is there a cup holder included or pocket? This is helpful for storing keys/phone/purse etc.

Some parents prefer a pram with the baby facing them rather than away from them. This enables you to chat to your baby as you walk along. Communicating with your baby constantly will aid her language development long term and encourage her to begin vocalising.

Something I also found very useful was being able to click the car seat on to my pushchair chassis. This meant that if I needed to pop into town in the car I was able to do this without having to transfer the baby from car seat into a pram/pushchair, and then back again, and most probably waking her if she had dozed off!

As this is a very practical item, the choice made will also need to be based on where you are planning to use it and for what purpose. Many large baby stores will be able to give advice and guide you on this.

I thoroughly enjoyed choosing the pram for my three children and had a different one for each of them. In fact, most people don't reuse them for subsequent babies as circumstances may have changed, so choose something based on your current needs and circumstances.

Important tip

Make sure the pushchair/pram that you do decide on actually fits into your car boot easily. As most will be home delivered by the shop, or come pre-packed in a big box that you transport home with your car's back seats down, you may not discover this until a later date. You don't want to use it a few times on walks round your local village, then plan an outing in the car and find that, when folded up, it doesn't fit! Also make sure that you know how to fold it before the baby is born as they can be surprisingly complicated to the uninitiated.

Car seat (essential)

Even if you don't own a car it's always advisable to buy a car seat. Some pushchairs come with them as part of the package, but if yours doesn't then you need to purchase or borrow one that's suitable for a newborn. You will need one to bring the baby home from the hospital anyway, and most maternity wards will not let you walk out with the baby in your arms. They generally ask your partner or family member to bring a car seat in on your day of discharge.

It is safer to buy a brand-new one so that you know it meets and has passed all of the current British safety standards. However, if you do choose to borrow one or purchase second-hand, only do so if you are certain that it has never been in a car that has been involved in an accident before. If you can't be sure of that then it's advisable to spend the extra money and buy a new one.

Some points to remember regarding car seats are:

- Never strap one into a passenger seat that has an active air bag. Turn the airbag off if you need to have the car seat in the front.
- Car seats for newborns are always rear-facing
- Get someone experienced to show you how to strap the car seat into the car correctly. Practise doing it before the baby is born so that you and your partner are both sure you know how to do it properly. Practice makes perfect!

I remember watching a friend strap her son, aged eight months into the car using both the rear passenger belt *and* the front passenger belt pulled into the back! She said she had been sitting in the back with the baby since he was born as she couldn't use the passenger seat in the front without use of the seat belt, which was being used for her son's car seat in the back! She couldn't stop laughing when I showed her the correct way to strap it in – using only one seat belt – and now enjoys car journeys sitting in the front with her husband, with the baby safely strapped in the back!

Baby carrier/sling (helpful)

This is another item that isn't essential but is very helpful to have around. If you are on a budget, it is probably something that you can try to borrow one from a friend to see how much you end up using it. It's a lifestyle item, really. If you enjoy going for long walks in the countryside, where a pushchair/pram may struggle over rough ground, then a baby carrier is a must-have item. Equally, if this isn't your first baby and you already have other children, then a sling can be very helpful in enabling you to carry a small baby around, but still have hands free on outings, or even to do jobs in the house if the baby is fretful in the early weeks.

The other great thing about slings is that they're fun, they promote bonding between you and your baby, and babies love them!

If you do decide you would like to make use of a sling, then a couple of things to look for are:

- That it's washable
- That the baby can be forward-facing or rear-facing
- That it has good neck support for a newborn

Baby monitors (essential)

A whole assortment of baby monitors can be found on the market. They range from a basic listening device, costing around £20–£30, which includes a baby unit for the nursery and a parent unit for you to hear them, to a more complex video and movement monitor, which can set you back around £200.

In my opinion the best type to go for would be a movement and sound baby monitor. This is what I used for all three of my children and the one I recommend to all of my clients who ask for advice. It is more expensive than a monitor that only registers noise, but well worth the extra money as it monitors your baby's breathing and buys peace of mind, which for most parents is priceless anyway. It comes with a movement mat that is placed under the mattress (cot or Moses basket), which will then cause an alarm to go off on the nursery unit and parent unit if it doesn't detect any movement for a certain amount of time. The sensitivity of the amount of movement picked up can be altered to the parents' preference.

There are a few different companies selling these types of monitors, ranging from £40–£100. Angelcare is the biggest brand name out there and the one I personally used with my children. It is also the one I recommend to all of the parents I work for. Contrary to popular belief, these monitors do not have the alarm going off all the time unnecessarily. The only time they begin to be pointless to use is when the baby begins to roll and move around the cot in her sleep. This means she rolls off and away from the mat, so the alarm will then go off as it's not detecting any movement. It varies from baby to baby and how much they move as to when you get to this stage. We had to stop using the Angelcare with our eldest son when he was five months as he kept rolling off the mat and setting the alarm off. However, for my other son and daughter we continued to use it until they were both over a year old, as they barely moved at all in their sleep and just stayed in the same position. Up until you reach this point, though, they are very effective and I found them to be very reassuring.

As a parent, cot death – or SIDS (sudden infant death syndrome) – is one of the main things you worry about, and you pray that your child will never be one of the unlucky ones (see also page 157). I loved the reassurance and security of something else 'keeping an eye on my baby', watching over her, in a way, while I slept. I trusted that the alarm would alert me if there was a problem, and I personally found that it made me feel a little more in control of the whole cot-death scenario. I thought that maybe, with the alarm to wake me where I otherwise may have still been sleeping, I may just be able to prevent the unthinkable happening if I were quick enough to get to my baby at the first signs of her not breathing. It is wise to enrol on a basic parent first-aid course before your baby is born or at least learn how to perform infant CPR so that you are aware of what to do if you did need to resuscitate your baby. Again you hope it will never be needed, but it is very reassuring to know the ropes.

These movement monitors are also particularly helpful and reassuring to use with premature babies, so it's helpful to have one of these in place for when you bring the baby home from hospital.

Breathing lapses are very common in premature babies: about 50 per cent of those born before 32 weeks' gestation experience them. Aponea monitors are used routinely in most special-care wards as premature babies can sometimes 'forget' to breathe every now and then when they are in a very deep sleep. Having the alarm means the staff are alerted to the baby. Most of the time all it takes is either a quick rub as they are snoozing, or to pick them up, which stimulates them enough to breathe regularly again.

This apnoea immaturity, when it occurs before the baby's original due date is totally unrelated to SIDS. It doesn't increase the risk of your baby succumbing to SIDS or to apnoea itself later on. If your baby continues to have serious and regular breathing issues after her original due date then contact your doctor. Brief lapses in breathing without any blueness or limpness or need for resuscitation, even in full-term babies, is not believed by most experts to be a predictor of SIDS risk, and most babies who do die of SIDS weren't observed to experience apnoea previously. Please see Chapter 5 for more details on causes and prevention of SIDS.

I don't really see the need for video monitoring if you have got the movement and sensor mat. You cannot tell if a baby is breathing or not just by looking at them sleeping on a small TV screen, but again it is down to individual preference.

Nursery furnishings and other useful items at home
Clothes storage (essential)
The type of wardrobe and/or chest of drawers you choose will very much depend on what built-in storage you already have in the nursery, and how much space you have left in the nursery once the cot is in place. It is helpful to have a set of drawers with a changing tabletop built on, where you can put your changing mat and be able to get the baby dressed without having to bend down on to the floor. This is especially helpful after a C-section.

Nursery chair (helpful)
Again this will depend on space available within the nursery, but if you can possibly squeeze one in then you will find it a godsend for those dreaded night feeds. Most come with a stool to put your feet up too; the one I had was so comfortable I used to walk past the nursery and find my husband dozing in it – without the baby!

There are so many different styles on the market, but try to find one that has arms as it makes breastfeeding your baby a lot easier. It can also be used to support your arm when bottle-feeding and later on as a chair you both snuggle up on for bedtime cuddles and story time.

Curtains and blackout blinds (essential)

It is vital to have both a fitted blackout blind that fits flush with the window and fully lined blackout curtains in the nursery. I know from 10 years' experience that having the room that the baby sleeps in as dark as you can possibly get it, with no chinks of light coming through, will make a huge difference to how well they sleep, both during their daytime naps and at night.

If you choose to have the baby in your room for the first few weeks then you also need to make sure that this room is made as dark as possible. All babies come into a light sleep from around 5 a.m. onwards. If they begin to stir and open their eyes and it is light enough in the room for them to see things, e.g., mobile, pictures, cuddly toys etc., they are more likely to wake fully. They may then find it hard to settle back to sleep until their normal 7–7:30 a.m. wake-up time. If, however, the room is so dark that they cannot make sense of any stimulating items in the room, then they are more likely just to doze back off to sleep again, and that means you can too! Blackout blinds, or material with sticky-back Velcro to place on the back of the blackout and then attach to the window, can be bought at many large department stores.

> **Tip**
> *Ensure there are no looped curtain cords that hang down where your baby may be able to reach them as she gets older, as these will carry a high risk of strangulation.*

Lighting (essential)

It's important to keep the lights very low for the night feeds, so as not to stimulate your baby too much or wake her fully. The aim will be to feed her and get her settled straight after, and the amount of lighting you use can affect how easily that happens. You will be able to control how well your baby settles, by adjusting the amount of stimulation and light she receives. If there isn't a dimmer fitted to the main light switch then it's a good idea to get one fitted. If this isn't possible then purchase a small lamp and put a 10- or 15-watt bulb in it, or buy a plug-in night light for the nursery to use when you breast- or bottle-feed your baby in the night.

Flooring/carpets (helpful)

A fitted carpet will help to keep the nursery warm in the wintertime. Try to avoid rugs as you may end up tripping over them during the night-time feeds, when the lights are low or off.

Baby bath (not needed)

This is not an essential item as the baby can very easily go into a big bath from day one. Baby baths themselves just tend to be another bulky item for which you will need to find space. They are also very difficult and heavy to try to empty out, unless you put them in the big bath – but then there isn't much point in having one if that's the case!

Bath aids (helpful)

There are a variety of bath aids on the market that are all very helpful in allowing you to have your hands free as you are bathing your baby. Newborns in particular tend to be very slippery as you are trying to handle them in the bath, so bath aids help to hold them in position while you gently splash water over them. The comfort of a bath aid also makes them feel a lot more reassured and secure so they are more likely to enjoy their bath from an early age. Smiling and chatting as you bathe her will also teach her from the start that bath time is a nice enjoyable experience with Mummy and/or Daddy.

I used a very basic towelling-type aid that looked like a mini-slide. It had a metal frame covered in towelling for the baby to lie on. You could wet the towel with the bath water before placing the baby on it to make it nice and warm for her. It could then be hooked on the inside of the bath to dry out when finished, ready for the next bath time.

Changing mat (helpful)

If you live over more than one storey, it's helpful to have two of these: one for upstairs and one for downstairs. That way you don't have to keep moving one whenever you need it. They are inexpensive and this can save a lot of running around in the first few weeks, which is particularly helpful as this is a time when your energy stores are low anyway. My current favourite is one with the slogan: 'Keep calm and change my bum!' Humour is always good when dealing with poo.

Bouncy chair/baby chair (helpful)

This is also a very helpful piece of equipment to have. Again there are many different types you can choose from, but some tips to help you choose the right one are below:

- Reclining chairs that can be altered to lie flat for a newborn and gradually raised to different heights as your baby grows and her neck gets stronger are very useful. These are also great if you have twins and need to use the chair to be able to feed both at the same time with a bottle.
- Choose one that has a 'head hugger' or neck support insert for when your baby is newborn and their head is still very floppy.
- Look for a chair that has a removable washable fabric. Wet wipes are great for wiping clean small spillages, but a large vomit or nappy explosion may mean the washing machine is the only place for it! Ensure you put it into some detergent to soak first if you are unable to put it straight into the washing machine.
- Choose one with straps. A newborn may not move a lot, but it's amazing how just wriggling around can mean they slide to the end of the chair if not strapped in. Always use the straps if you are going to be leaving the room for any period of time.

- Consider attached toys. It isn't essential to have one with these, as many people tend to buy a baby gym of sorts anyway. This can then be placed over the chair for the baby to look up at the toys and eventually reach out to play with.

Musical or vibrating chairs and swinging chairs are not a necessity and can be very expensive. As long as you have a standard baby chair and some toys, even if separate from the chair, it will be enough.

Baby gym/play mat/rattles (helpful)

Again, there are lots to choose from but I found the most practical was a play mat with a curved frame that you attached, which then had various toys hanging down. These can be folded away easily and packed into a bag, and taken on holiday or to grandparents' etc. The toys are detachable so as the baby gets older you are able to take them off the main frame and give them to her to chew on and explore while she sits in her bouncy chair. Alternatively the bouncy chair can be sat on the play mat, so that the baby can reach the attached toys hanging down. They can also lie directly on the mat under the toys to reach up to them.

Other extras

A **baby thermometer** is a good thing to have in the house just in case your baby seems unwell. Choose a digital one as they are the most accurate, easy to use and read, and give a fast reading. The most common digital thermometers are underarm ones or ones where the reading is taken in the ear. Rectal digital thermometers can also be bought, although most parents do not like the idea of taking their baby's temperature in this way. The underarm ones are the cheaper to buy of the two, costing less than £10, and in my opinion are the most accurate. An ear thermometer will set you back a bit more, costing somewhere between £20 and £60 depending on what brand you get, although they are not recommended for babies younger than six months because their narrow ear canals make it difficult to get an accurate reading.

Nail scissors are also good to have on hand. It always amazes me how long and sharp babies' nails are even at birth. They are able to do themselves some real damage clawing at their own faces as they try to eat their hands when hungry or for comfort, so it's important to make sure that you check them every couple of days, and trim or cut them when necessary. Babies' nails are very soft so sometimes you will be able to nibble at them with your own teeth to keep them short; in fact, some people swear by this method and never need to use scissors. I've found a bit of both works, and, after trying many different types of baby clippers and scissors, the Tommee Tippee ones are the easiest to use in my opinion.

Baby hairbrushes with the soft bristles are helpful to have, particularly if your baby has lots of hair. If your baby is born with barely any hair then you may not need to use one initially but it will still come in handy later.

Large baby stores or department stores tend to sell a **complete baby health and grooming kit**, which will contain all of the above, as well as medicine droppers and various other items depending on where you buy it. This is likely to be the cheapest option.

There are many other items and equipment available to buy but I have tried to give you some basis to begin with on items that will be necessary to have from the start. You may also find other things that are really helpful to fit your lifestyle. Your first baby is a real learning curve, and you realise what things are important to have around and what is not, purely by experiencing the first year with your baby. This will then give you more of an idea of what you need, can reuse or replace if/when you have subsequent children.

Nappies, wipes and cotton pads (essential)
It's a personal choice as to whether to go for cloth/reusable nappies or disposable ones. If you would like to use cloth nappies

then there are nappy services available that will collect your soiled nappies, take them away and bring them back clean to save you the job of doing it, which can make life easier.

There are many different brands of disposable nappies. During the first few weeks it's normal for your baby to have 6–10 soiled nappies per day, so buying nappies can be very expensive as you will go through so many. I purchased a cheaper supermarket brand to put on my babies during the day, as they were never wearing them for any length of time. It's wise to use a more expensive premium brand of nappy at night-time though, as they will be less likely to leak, and less likely to require a whole outfit change at 4 a.m.!

Navigating nappies

- *If you have a boy, always ensure his penis is pointing down before you do his nappy up. The nappy is much more likely to leak if you don't.*

- *A disposable nappy needs to be done up quite tightly with no gaps at the sides to prevent leakages. As long as you can place two fingers down the front of the nappy where your baby's tummy button is then it won't be too tight. In fact, most nappies are elasticated so it's virtually impossible to do it up too tight.*

- *There is also a 'lip' that runs round each of your baby's legs once the nappy is done up. Ensure that this isn't tucked in or the nappy will also be more likely to leak.*

- *Use fragrance-free wipes as they are kinder to your baby's bottom than the perfumed wipes. Some babies are very sensitive to wet wipes for the first few months and will come out in a rash if you use them on their bottom. It is generally something they grow out of as their skin gets more acclimatised to all the bacteria in the air.*

- *Cotton pads are better to use than cotton wool balls, as they are not fluffy and don't fall apart when you start wiping. Use the pads* with warm water and pat your baby's bottom dry afterwards before putting a clean nappy on her.

- Talcum powder is not essential to use, even after a bath. It may make your baby smell nice but doesn't allow the skin to breathe and can cause rashes in babies with more sensitive skin.

- Nappy rash cream like Sudocrem and Metanium are good to use when your baby has a red or sore bottom. I would not advise using them every time you change your baby's nappy, the cream manufacturers may encourage you to do this as a means to sell more, but it is more effective if you only use it when needed. Apply a small amount to your baby's dry bottom on the rash or red areas. Rub it in using circular motions until it is almost invisible. In the case of cream for nappy rash, less is more! Do not be tempted to apply lashings of cream as this will possibly make the rash or redness worse, as the cream sitting on top of your baby's skin will go on to the nappy and prevent it effectively absorbing your baby's urine. This urine will then be wet on your baby's bottom and make her even more sore.

Equipment needed for breastfeeding

Breast pump (essential)

You have the option of a manual or electric breast pump and even single or double ones. In my experience it has been down to the preference of the mother. My view was that I already felt like a bit of a milked cow anyway, so I didn't fancy adding to that feeling by attaching myself to something electric that did the pumping for me! As a result I opted for a manual breast pump. Other women may find the idea of not pumping manually very appealing as it saves them the effort. Each to their own.

It's a good idea to buy a breast pump that is the same make as your bottles. That way your pump will fit directly on to your baby's bottles. Once you have 'pumped', all you then need to do is put a sterilised teat on the expressed bottle of milk and leave in the fridge ready to use if you need it. Alternatively, you can freeze any excess milk that you don't feed to the baby immediately.

Freezer bags (essential)

These are an essential buy when breastfeeding as you will quickly develop the attitude that no breast milk at all should be wasted, no matter how little you manage to pump off and save. You need to buy specialised freezer bags made purely for storing breast milk. They will come ready-sterile in boxes of 20 or 40. Your excess breast milk can be poured directly into one of these bags, sealed and then placed in your freezer and stored for up to six months. They can be purchased from some large supermarkets, but you'll also find them in large pharmacy chains or your local baby department store.

Nursing pillow (essential)

A good nursing pillow makes the world of difference when breastfeeding. Due to the amount of time you will be sitting down feeding the baby it is so important to find a comfortable support that will enable you to find good feeding positions. I have seen many different-shaped pillows and cushions, but the one I would recommend to use is the V-shaped pillow. Make sure you buy one that is a bit squashy and not completely firm, and also has a washable cover to go over the actual pillow. I bought mine very cheaply (less than £15), brand new, off a major auction site.

It can also have many other uses apart from being used as a breastfeeding pillow. Other uses include:

- Support for your bump when pregnant. You can sleep with it tucked around your bump and between your legs when lying on your side to make yourself more comfortable.
- 'A safety pillow' when your baby is a bit older and learning to sit up, but not quite steady enough to leave without cushions around to catch her. You can put it behind her so that she will have a soft landing should she topple over.

- Somewhere to lie Baby down but propped up after a feed, particularly if the bouncy chair isn't available. It is never a good idea to lay a baby flat on their back immediately after a feed, because if there is still some remaining wind this will cause her to be sick! Once she seems relaxed on the cushion for 10 minutes or so with no further wriggling, you can then transfer her to the Moses basket or cot.

Nipple creams (helpful)

If your baby is positioned correctly from the start and never allowed to suck for long periods on an empty breast, then the hope is that you will never need to use nipple creams or sprays. As discussed in Chapter 4 in the feeding section, if you gradually build up the time that the baby has on the breast, then your nipples will have time to get used to being sucked.

The reason a lot of women tend to get bleeding and cracked nipples is because the newborn baby is allowed to suck for long periods of time in the first couple of days. As you are only producing tiny amounts of colostrum for the first two to five days before your full milk supply begins to come in and build up, the only thing you will achieve is getting sore nipples very quickly! Once you have sore, cracked or bleeding nipples it is very difficult to get them back in good shape again. The baby will continue to feed, even more so once your milk comes in, so your breasts will never get a long enough period of time to rest and recover.

Dummies are a godsend in the first few days before your milk comes in, to allow the breast to get used to feeding gradually. (See page 29 for more information on dummies).

Tips to prevent sore/cracked nipples:

- Initially feed for 10–15 minutes on each side only and build up to a maximum of 30 minutes on any one side once your milk comes in.

- The small bumps on the areola (dark area surrounding your nipple) are called Montgomery glands. They produce natural oil that cleans, lubricates and protects the nipple during pregnancy and breastfeeding. This oil contains an enzyme that kills bacteria and makes breast creams unnecessary for a lot of women. Use only water to clean your breasts. Soaps, lotions or alcohol-based products may remove this protective oil.

- Check the baby is positioned correctly on the breast. You should feel her sucking and pulling at the breast as she feeds but it shouldn't be a painful experience the whole time she is on there. When your milk comes in around days three to five you will find that the latching-on process *is* teeth-grindingly painful for about the first 10–15 seconds. This is very normal, and once you get your 'let down' of milk flowing, the pain passes and the pulling/sucking sensation resumes! This initial latching-on pain isn't something that is widely discussed – women are constantly told that if it hurts then the baby is not positioned correctly. While that is correct on the whole, it is very normal for women to experience the latching-on pain. I had it with all three of my babies, all my friends who breastfed experienced it too, and all the mums I work for are the same. Unfortunately it is part and parcel of establishing breastfeeding. It may happen every time your baby latches on, even if she falls off and you have to put her back on again. It is like very bad pins and needles in your nipple and lasts for around 10–15 seconds, at which point you will gradually feel the pain fade away. If it remains painful after the first 15 seconds, though, then you need to take the baby off the breast and try the latching-on process again, as it's likely that she doesn't have enough of the areola in her mouth and is possibly just chomping on your nipple.

In my opinion the reason a lot of women give up breastfeeding in the first few weeks is because they are not informed of this latching-on pain. They think they must be doing something wrong as they are experiencing this pain every time, and all the literature is telling them that pain means the baby is not latched on correctly. They are then more likely to break the baby off the breast straight away, rather than persevering through the first 15 seconds of pain, as nobody has informed them that it is normal for all of us!

If after doing all of the above you still get sore or cracked nipples then you can try some cream to relieve the pain. The product that in my opinion is the best by far is made by a company called Lansinoh. It is more expensive than most but it is the leading lanolin cream for sore nipples and cracked skin. It's 100 per cent natural and has no additives, preservatives or chemicals, and the most wonderful thing about it is you don't need to wash it off before breastfeeding. It is safe for your baby and they don't even mind or notice the taste.

I was very lucky and never needed to use any nipple creams etc., but I bought this cream when my eight-month-old had dry/cracked skin on her thumb that she constantly sucked. I was worried her thumb would get infected if I left it, but I knew I needed to find a cream that was safe for her to still suck her thumb once applied. The Lansinoh was perfect. I put it on her thumb three or four times per day and within a couple of days her thumb was back to its normal self. She was even very happy to pop her thumb in her mouth immediately after an application of it and not show any signs of being unhappy about the taste!

Other mums have also used Lansinoh for nappy rash, itchy stretch marks, minor cuts, burns or abrasions, dry skin patches and as a naturally moisturising lip balm!

Breast pads (essential)

These are essential for when your milk comes in. Some mothers do not tend to leak once their breasts settle down a few days after the milk first comes in; others will soak through breast pads and have to change them every hour! Both scenarios are normal and even if you don't have so much milk that you leak you should still be able to breastfeed successfully.

Dummies (essential)

I believe that dummies are essential in the early weeks of having a new baby, whether you breastfeed or bottle-feed. If used correctly and at the right times, there will never be an issue of the baby becoming so attached and dependent on them that it's then upsetting to wean them.

Recent studies also reported a lower SIDS (sudden infant death syndrome, or cot death) incidence among infants who use a dummy, although more research needs to be done to confirm these findings. See Chapter 5 for more information on SIDS.

Newborn babies tend to like having something to suck for comfort when agitated. In the early days they will root around almost constantly when awake, and not settle until something is put into their mouth! If you are breastfeeding and trying not to use the dummy, this will mean you end up putting them to the breast to calm them down. With only a minimal amount of colostrum in your breasts until your full milk supply comes in, the baby will end up sucking on an empty breast regularly. This will mean your nipples will not have time to get used to the art of breastfeeding and you will get sore very quickly.

Using a dummy in the early days will *not* put your baby off the breast or affect how quickly you get feeding established as some books and so-called experts suggest! I have used a dummy with every single baby I have worked with, 90 per cent of whom are breastfed in the beginning, as well as with all three of my own children, and never had any problems getting any of them established on the breast. Dummies are very helpful in enabling you to work out if your baby is genuinely hungry or just looking for a bit of comfort.

The trick is to offer a dummy when your baby is rooting around looking like she is hungry. Usually if it is just a bit of comfort sucking she is looking for then she will latch on to it straight away, calm down and be more settled. Persevere for five to ten minutes if she doesn't take the dummy immediately. Tease her with the teat of the dummy as she roots around, and let her suck the dummy into her mouth fully. If you just push the dummy straight into her mouth she is likely to gag, so you need to let her draw it into her mouth rather than forcing it straight in.

If she does calm down straight away and relaxes then you have given her some comfort in using the dummy and stalled the feed a bit longer, which means she is more likely to take a bigger feed at the guide time. That is ultimately what you are trying to achieve. If you feed a baby every time they root around because you don't have a dummy to use, then very quickly you will end up with a snack feeder who only ever takes a small feed because they are feeding so often! They will then understandably need to feed a short time later because they didn't feed for long enough and get the right balance of fore milk/hind milk to be able to sustain themselves. This is explained in more detail in the feeding section – see Chapter 4. If after persevering with the dummy for 10 minutes the baby is still rooting around and crying, then indications are that she is genuinely hungry and the dummy will not sustain a hungry baby who is desperate for a feed. See the feeding section for what to do in this instance.

Dummies should never be used as a sleep prop. If you always give your baby a dummy to get her to sleep, and allow her to suck it while asleep, she will become dependent on it very quickly. She will then begin to wake up and look for it every time she comes into a light sleep and realises it has fallen out of her mouth. This will mean you having to get up and replace it constantly every night – clearly not a great habit to get into.

If, after a feed, your baby is very unsettled, doesn't want to feed any more, is not showing signs of obvious wind, and is still wide-awake when she should really be going back to sleep, you can use the dummy to get her drowsy. She will not learn to rely on the dummy if you always make sure you remove it before she drops into a deep sleep. Let her suck on it in a darkened room until she is looking very sleepy and then gently remove it. If she starts fretting and begins to wake again fully then put it back in her mouth and then try to remove it again a few minutes later. Sometimes you will manage to take it away first time, or you may have to do this two or three times. The main thing is that a baby is not allowed to keep sucking it while asleep as this will be where the dependency problems begin!

It's advisable to dispose of all current dummies after one month of use and replace with new ones.

Equipment needed for bottle-feeding
Steriliser (essential)
This is a must-have, essential item when bottle-feeding. Its purpose is to kill germs on your baby's feeding equipment in order to keep your baby healthy. It's also good to have one if breastfeeding too as the breast pump, dummies, etc. will also need to be sterilised once in use.

An alternative option for sterilising is to buying Milton sterilising tablets. Use them as directed on the packaging with cold water and soak all feeding bottles, teats, dummies, etc. for a minimum of two hours. This was the method used years ago before steam sterilisers were invented.

Steam sterilisers are easier but it is worth having a packet of Milton tablets in the cupboard just in case your steam steriliser should fail at any point. It would be bad luck for it to happen at 10 p.m. one night for example, as you are hoping for a good night's sleep and need to make up the following day's bottles.

In my experience a steam steriliser is the fastest, easiest and most practical way of keeping your feeding equipment clean, germ-free and sterile. You have the option of buying a free-standing electric steam steriliser or a microwave steam steriliser. There are various brands of both, and both take five to ten minutes to run their sterilising process. Electric steam sterilisers tend to be able to fit six bottles compared to a microwave steriliser, which can fit four bottles in. You will also need to buy specific de-scaling sachets. The steriliser will need de-scaling every four to six weeks to keep it working effectively.

It's advisable to buy the same brand steriliser as your bottle choice to ensure they will fit, and most companies will have a package of steriliser and bottles that you can buy together.

Bottles (essential)

With so many different brands to choose from it's hard to know which bottles to choose. Each company claims that their bottle is the best one to prevent colic, wind, etc. I have tried and tested all of the brands. Over the years I have worked with hundreds of babies and my recommendation to anyone who asks for my opinion is to go for the Philips AVENT range. They sell a wide-necked, anti-colic, BPA-free bottle and that has been my favoured option.

BPA stands for bisphenol A, a substance that is included in all polycarbonate products like baby bottles and other containers made for everyday use around the home. Recent health scares concerning polycarbonate baby bottles containing bisphenol A centre around a report produced in the USA, which claims that long-term exposure to BPA *could* result in health and developmental implications for infants and children. The concern is that in preparing a bottle by heating to a high temperature in a steriliser and/or microwave, babies could ingest a small quantity of BPA, which leaks out of polycarbonate bottles more easily if they have been heated to a high temperature. There is, as yet, no long-term research or evidence to support a major health scare, and the latest report from the US National Institutes of Health puts their alert level midway between low and high and advises 'some concern'.

The current advice for concerned parents who are bottle-feeding is to either switch to glass bottles *or* use a hot water-filled jug or bottle warmer to heat existing polycarbonate bottles *or* switch to one of the many BPA-free bottles now available in the UK. Most of the leading bottle or cup manufacturers, including Tommee Tippee, Philips AVENT, MAM, Medela, Mothercare and NUK, offer BPA-free bottles and cups that are available from most leading supermarkets and independent pharmacies. Further information on their BPA-free ranges can be obtained from their websites.

This scare happened after both my boys had already used bottles containing BPA, as it did with many other parents and babies. We are unable to change what effect it may or may not have had on the children who have already been subjected to it. As a parent about to buy new bottles for your baby, I would advise you to purchase the BPA-free bottles, which is what I did for my daughter, who was born after this health scare. At least it will give you one less thing to worry about!

Teats (essential)

Most bottles come with a slow-flow teat, or number 1. This will be engraved into the teat so you can see the number. Most brands of bottles have numbered teats that have faster and increased milk flow the higher number teat you use. Generally they go up to a size 3 or 4.

For a newborn baby you would start off with a number 1 teat initially. If they don't seem to be taking much at each feed, it's always worth trying them on the next size up teat, even if they are younger than the age recommended on the packaging. Try the faster-flow teat over two or three feeds to see if that makes a difference to the amount of milk they take.

Another indicator that you need to move your baby to a faster-flow teat as they get older will be if they start to decrease the amount they take at each feed, or fall asleep. This usually happens because they become bored of having to work hard on a slow teat once they get a bit bigger and have a stronger suck. They will take an initial amount to satisfy their immediate hunger, but then usually when you stop to wind them, they will refuse to make the effort to take any more, as it's just too much like hard work! Moving up a teat size should encourage your baby to increase the amount they take at each feed.

Most breastfed babies who are introduced to a bottle of expressed milk or formula from a few weeks old tend to move up to a number 2 teat very quickly. This is because they are so used to controlling the flow of milk from the breast and they find a number 1 teat too slow.

Bottlebrush, dishwashing liquid and bowl (essential)

You will need to buy a bottlebrush that is to be used solely for cleaning all of the baby's feeding equipment. These can easily be found in the baby aisle of any major supermarket. Bottles and feeding equipment should be soaked in a bowl of hot, soapy water, cleaned with a bottlebrush thoroughly and then the bubbles rinsed out using cold or hot water. They can then be placed in your steriliser.

Bottle warmer (helpful)

This is not essential, but can be very useful if you don't have or want to use a microwave to heat feeds. It is also much faster than boiling a kettle full of water and then standing the bottle in hot water to heat.

Equally it is not essential to heat formula feeds. If you are using the ready-made cartons then the baby can have them at room temperature. You can easily pour the carton contents into a sterile bottle and feed immediately.

However, most parents who formula-feed their babies solely tend to buy the large tubs of powdered milk as it's a much cheaper option. As you will probably be making up feeds in advance, you will need to heat them a little at least to take the chill off the milk where it has been stored in the fridge.

If you do need to heat the feed it is okay to use a microwave. (90 per cent of the parents I work for choose to heat their baby's feed this way – it is certainly fastest.) Unscrew the lid off the top and put just the bottle itself in the microwave to heat the milk. Replace the lid. As long as you ensure that you shake the bottle thoroughly after heating then you won't get any 'hotspots' in the milk, which concerns some people. After shaking the milk you then need to test the temperature to make sure it is okay to give to your baby.

A bottle warmer is also another fast way of heating milk – speed is always of the essence at 3 a.m. when you have a crying, hungry baby! It's always best to buy the same brand bottle warmer as the bottles that you plan to use. This will ensure that your bottles actually fit in.

Alternatively, as mentioned above, the old-fashioned way of boiling the kettle and then pouring some hot water into a jug or bowl and standing the bottle in it is still effective.

Clothes needed in the beginning

With so many cute outfits lining the shelves of baby stores and supermarkets these days, it's very easy to spend a lot of money on clothes that your baby will barely wear at all before she grows out of them. You are also likely to get lots of baby-grows as presents from family and friends. You, like all other parents-to-be, will be unable to resist some outfits, but below I have compiled a list of clothing and items that will be essential to have for everyday use.

Sizing

Most newborn-sized clothes only fit babies up to around 9–10lb (4–4.5kg) in weight. If your baby is born at this weight then they will not fit into newborn clothes and will go straight into the 0–3 month size. It's best to pack one size of each in your hospital bag, just in case, as you won't know how big your baby will be until she is born.

Vests and baby-grows

These are perfect in the first few weeks for both day and night wear. Try to buy ones made of 100 per cent cotton. This is the best fabric for her to wear to prevent her getting too hot or coming out in a rash. The type that fastens using press-studs at the bottom, rather than with ties, is the best. These ones are easier to put on when getting her dressed and, with the press studs fastening under her nappy, you have easy access to change it, without having to completely undress her every time. They can be bought in packs of three or more, and come in various colours.

Scratch mitts

These are little gloves that go over your baby's hands to prevent her scratching herself. I think they are essential in the first few weeks until your baby develops a little more awareness of her hands. Her nails will be very sharp, even from day one, and babies tend to claw at their faces when rooting around and trying to eat their hands in the search for milk. Scratch mitts are particularly useful at night, but sometimes need to be used during the day for babies that are determined to attack their own faces at every opportunity as soon as their hands are freed! Many baby-grows now sold in the shops have these built into them, and you can fold them over your baby's hands so that they won't slip off.

Bibs

These are to use during feeding, particularly for those babies that are bottle-fed, but it's very helpful to have a supply of bibs even if you plan on breastfeeding. They are great for catching any vomit or possetting after a feed, preventing an entire outfit change. The plastic-backed ones tend to be better, as any milk that goes on to an entirely material based bib will seep through on to your babies outfit anyway, defeating the purpose of using a bib in the first place.

> **Tip**
> **Always remove bibs** before putting your baby down for a nap to prevent the risk of strangulation as she moves around in her sleep.

Muslin squares

These can be bought in packs in various colours and are fantastic as a shield for your clothes. They are made of 100 per cent cotton, square-shaped, and in terms of thickness are between a handkerchief and a cot sheet. They are fantastic for putting over your shoulder when winding your baby to protect your clothes from the inevitable possetting or even vomit that may come out with your baby's burps, which otherwise end up all over your clothes. I always make sure that I have a muslin draped over my shoulder whenever I carry a small baby around. It's best to be prepared! They are easy to wash and dry and can also later be used as a sleep comforter once you no longer swaddle your baby. (See Chapter 5 for more details.)

Socks

These can be worn under baby-grows on cold winter nights and with day clothes.

Cardigans

You can be sure that well-meaning relatives will donate plenty of these to you. I got so many I didn't know what to do with them all, and my mum still gives me a new one for my little girl almost every time I see her.

They are useful in the early weeks for day use to put over the top of her vest and baby-grow to keep her warm on a chilly day. I wouldn't recommend using a cardigan at night, particularly when your baby is swaddled, as you don't want her to overheat.

Day clothes

As mentioned, there is such a wide range of fashionable outfits you can buy for your baby to dress them up like little adults. Day clothes are not essential in the first few weeks as you can just use a change of vest and baby-grow. However, it is nice to have a few special outfits all prepared for when Granny comes to visit! Stick mainly to buying the 0–3 month size or bigger, as you will find that you barely get any use out of the newborn-sized clothes.

Coat/all-in-one suit

Depending on what time of the year your baby is due to be born, just buying a warm coat may be sufficient. However, if your baby is due in the winter then you will need to buy an all-in-one coat suit. These are generally made of a fleece or wool type of material, and have feet, mittens and a hood to keep your baby nice and snug.

Blankets/sheets/sleeping bags

There are various blankets and sheets you will need. I have listed a minimum amount to allow for washing etc.:

- **For cot/cot bed**: two cotton-jersey fitted sheets. The knitted construction of these sheets helps them to stretch easily and fit snug to the mattress. They are made from an easy-care material making them stress-free to wash and iron, and come in a range of colours.
- **For Moses basket**: two fitted sheets. The decorative bedding that can be bought with a Moses basket is not essential and down to parents' choice if you would like to buy it or not.
- **Three large cotton cellular blankets**: these are great for swaddling as the cellular construction of the blanket offers insulation as well as breathability, which is perfect for keeping your baby at the correct temperature. Fleece blankets are very popular but cellular blankets are safer, particularly at night-time.

- **Sleeping bag/grobag**: these come in various tog ratings from 0.5–2.5 so can be used all year round. You can use the lightweight bag for the warmer weather, and just dress your baby in a vest, and buy the thicker grobag for the winter. There are various styles, with or without sleeves, and they have a zip along the bottom, making night-time nappy changes easier.

Once you stop swaddling your baby it is a good idea to get her used to a sleeping bag straight away for all sleeps in the cot, during the day as well as night-time. Unlike blankets, a sleeping bag allows your baby to move freely without the risk of getting caught under the covers. This is something you need to be particularly conscious of once she begins rolling and even crawling. I've never used blankets in the basket or cot at night-time once my babies begin to roll and move around. Having a sleeping bag with the correct tog rating and dressing her in enough clothing will keep your baby warm but also prevent her crawling under the covers and becoming stuck. Using a sleeping bag also means that she can't kick off any bedcovers and then wake up feeling cold.

2

Going into hospital

As mentioned previously, it is best to pack your and the baby's items that will be needed into a bag a few weeks before your due date. I would recommend having it ready as early as 32 weeks, as it is so much nicer to be prepared in an emergency situation rather than relying on a partner or family member to get everything needed and bring to the hospital at a later stage. Only you really know what you want to have in it.

What to pack in your hospital bag
Below I have compiled one list for the baby and one list for items you will/may need. Some of the things on the Mummy list may not even get used, but it's best to have them in your bag just in case. You can always pass them on to a friend if you don't end up using them.

Baby items
- 1 pack of nappies
- 1 pack of wet wipes
- Cotton wool pads
- Nappy sacks
- 3 vests
- 3 baby-grows
- 1 pair of scratch mitts
- 2 bibs

- 2 muslin squares
- Newborn-size hat
- Bottles and formula if you are not breastfeeding.

Although you may only plan on staying in hospital for a few hours after the birth and then getting back home as soon as possible (all being well, of course), even that will be enough time for your newborn to wee or poo on more than one vest/baby-grow, so packing a few is essential. Usually a newborn size will be the correct one for most babies that are born, but be prepared that if your baby weighs over 9lb (4kg) at birth then she may not fit into it! I had this problem with my first son, and had to get my mum to take a detour on the way to the hospital to buy some bigger baby-grows to put him in. It's advisable to pack at least one vest and baby-grow in a 0–3-month size.

Mummy items
- Birthing nightshirt
- Cotton dressing gown. Go for a thin one as hospitals are kept at warm temperatures!
- 2 clean nightshirts for use after birth, with buttons or front opening if you plan on breastfeeding.
- 2 pairs of knickers
- 1 pack of large disposable knickers. These are fab to use in the first few days after birth when you are bleeding heavily, as they can just be thrown away if stained with blood. They are also great if you end up having a C-section as they can just be cut off, which saves you painfully bending down.
- 1 pack of maternity sanitary towels
- 1 pack of breast pads, although you shouldn't actually need these until your full milk supply comes in around day three after birth. It depends how long you end up having to stay in hospital.
- 2 breastfeeding bras if you plan on breastfeeding.

- Slippers
- Dettol wipes/hand sanitiser. This is usually provided, but it's always nice to have your own!
- Your birth plan
- Your maternity notes
- Camera, phone and chargers
- A notebook and pen
- Wash bag containing toothbrush, toothpaste, shower soap, deodorant and anything else you like.
- Small change for hospital car park or pay phone
- Day clothes to go home in when you are discharged

What to expect during labour and birth
Birth plans

It is a good idea to make a birth plan with your preferences in terms of labour positions, any pain relief you are happy to have and what you would like to happen after the baby is born. You can find examples on the NHS website to give you an idea of what information is needed. http://www.nhs.uk/conditions/pregnancy-and-baby/pages/birth-plan.aspx#close

Typically the topics you will need to cover in your birth plan are:

- Where you would like your baby to be born – at home or in hospital
- Pain relief you are happy to use during labour
- Special requests – use of birth pool for example
- Who will be present with you during the birth
- Your feelings about assisted delivery – forceps, ventouse, episiotomy, etc.
- Your wishes after birth regarding placenta delivery, who Baby is given to after birth, etc.

Pack your birth plan into your hospital bag and make sure your midwife is aware of it when you arrive. It can be kept with your maternity notes that you hand to her on arrival.

The biggest piece of advice I can give you about labour and giving birth, after having three children of my own, is to expect the unexpected and be prepared for your birth plan to change at short notice.

None of us know how we are going to react to the circumstances and pain that is involved with labour and giving birth. We all know what we would like to happen: that we will go through labour quickly and easily without any pain relief at all, and give birth to a healthy baby without batting an eyelid! However, we all have different pain thresholds, and none of us knows how our body will cope with labour, particularly first time round. In terms of pain relief it is best to just see what happens and go with the flow a bit. You will know if and when you get to the point of needing some form of pain relief, either to just take the edge off the pain or remove it all together.

I made a birth plan with my first baby stating that I would be happy to use the TENS machine at the start and then gas and air if the pain became too much. I also specified that I would prefer not to have pethidine or an epidural at all. I ended up having two doses of pethidine, an epidural and an emergency C-section after 14 hours in active labour, six of those stuck at 9.5cm dilated with contractions every two minutes! Needless to say, I didn't even bother making a birth plan for my next two children! Your instincts over what you want and need at the time will take over and get you through it all.

You haven't failed if you don't stick to your original birth plan; you have simply adapted to the circumstances surrounding you at the time. There are no prizes for going through all that pain with no help. The important thing is that you and the baby come out of it healthy and relatively unscathed at the end.

The mind forgets the pain

*Obviously, labour can be very intense and painful. I was so shocked as I looked down at my firstborn a couple of hours after he was born and thought, 'That was so awful that I am **never** doing that again.' At the time I was sure that I meant it without any doubt! I felt so sad looking at my baby boy thinking that he would have to now be an only child as I wasn't prepared to go through that type of experience again, when previous to my labour I had always said I wanted at least two children. It is amazing how quickly the mind forgets though, as just one month later I was saying, 'Well, when we have the next one…' much to my husband's surprise, who thought we were stopping at one!*

I have found the scenario I just described is normal for every new mum I have talked to. We all go through a few days or weeks after the birth resolutely stating that we will not have any more children, but most mums tend to change their minds. Nobody warned me of these feelings and they terrified me as I felt so strongly about it at that moment in time, and determined that I would never have another child. I also felt very sad at the same time. Because of this, I always try to warn friends and clients that this will be a perfectly normal feeling to have straight after your baby is born, and that, for most of us, it won't last! As painful as labour and birth is, our babies and children bring such love and joy to our lives from the day they are born that any amount of pain is worthwhile!

C-sections, ventouse and forceps delivery

As much as we all pray for a straightforward labour or birth, this is not really something that can be planned ahead.

Around one in eight women has an assisted birth, where forceps or a ventouse suction cup are used to help deliver the baby's head. This can be because:

- The baby is in an awkward position
- There are concerns labour is not progressing as well or as quickly as they would like and the baby's heart rate is abnormal
- The mum is too exhausted and needs a little help to make delivery easier

Both ventouse and forceps assistance are considered safe by the NHS and are only used when necessary for you and your baby.

If you have had problems in pregnancy and are already booked in for a Caesarean section, then you should have already been given all of the information and facts about how and when it will happen, and what is involved. It is a good idea to ensure you have a family member or friend who can step up and help out with childcare if you already have other children in the event that you have to stay in hospital longer than planned. Always pack your hospital bag to cater for at least one overnight stay, and make sure that your partner or someone else knows where to find any extra items that may need to be brought to hospital for you or the baby if needed. Don't be afraid to ask questions at your antenatal appointments about things you may be concerned about.

Breast- or bottle-feeding

If you plan on breastfeeding then you won't need to take anything into hospital in terms of feeding equipment. As mentioned in the hospital bag items list, just ensure that you pack a couple of nursing bras and some nightshirts that open at the front easily.

If your choice is to bottle-feed your baby, then you will most likely need to take bottles and some cartons to the hospital with you, as most maternity wards do not provide them any more. Check with your midwife to be sure. The ward will have a room (usually called the 'milk kitchen'), where you will be able to sterilise and make up your baby's bottles until you are discharged.

The first five things to expect after your baby arrives

1. Apgar score

The Apgar score is a quick test performed on a baby by a midwife or doctor at one minute and then at five minutes after birth. The one-minute score determines how the baby tolerated the birthing process and the five-minute score tells the doctors how well the baby is doing outside of the womb. It is sometimes repeated at 10 minutes if the baby's initial scores weren't good. The Apgar rating is based on an overall score of 1 to 10. Your baby's breathing effort, skin colour, heart rate, muscle tone and reflexes are all examined and each is given a score of 0, 1 or 2 depending on their condition, and then all are added up at the end. The higher the score, the better the baby is doing. A score of 7, 8 or 9 is normal and a sign that your baby is in good health. A score of 10 is very unusual as almost all newborns lose a point for blue hands and feet – both of which are completely normal after birth. Any score lower than 7 is a sign that the baby needs medical attention, and she may receive oxygen and need to have her airway cleared to help her breathe or physical stimulation to get her heart beating at a healthy rate. Most of the time a low score at one minute becomes near normal by five minutes. A lower Apgar score does not mean a child will have serious or long-term health problems and is not designed to predict the future health of the child. It is generally just caused by a difficult birth, a C-section or fluid in the baby's airway.

2. Meconium

This is the first bowel movement that your baby will pass. It is a greeny-black substance composed of materials ingested while your baby is inside you – cells, mucus, bile and water. It is very sticky and tar-like, which makes it very difficult to clean off your baby's bottom even with wet wipes! It has usually completely passed through her system after a couple of days, when her poo will begin to change to yellow in colour. This is a good indication that your milk is beginning to come through if you are breastfeeding.

Usually this substance is not released in your baby's bowel movements until after the birth. Occasionally though some babies will pass meconium while you are in labour. This will show itself in your waters as they break as they will be stained green instead of clear. If meconium is found to be present in your waters, then you will be monitored more closely, to check for foetal distress, and action will be taken if there is a problem. More often than not, babies who pass a small amount of meconium while the mother is in labour are born without any health issues – my eldest was one of these. My waters were stained green when they broke. I was put on a foetal monitor for the rest of my 14-hour labour, but luckily my baby boy was born healthy. In rare occasions a baby can ingest the meconium into their lungs while still in the womb, and this is a problem requiring medical attention.

3. Afterpains

Most women don't feel these after their first pregnancy and birth but will experience them with any subsequent children. Afterpains are caused by your uterus contracting as it attempts to shrink back to its pre-pregnancy size. It does this more efficiently after your first pregnancy, but your uterus loses muscle tone during subsequent pregnancies and it has to contract more, which is why it is felt more. The pain is very similar to period pain and you will feel cramping in your abdomen. If you decide to breastfeed you will feel the cramps more strongly as your baby latches on to feed. This is because your baby's sucking releases a hormone called oxytocin, which stimulates your uterus to contract more. If you do experience afterpains mention them to your midwife, and she will advise you on safe pain-relief medications. They will be most intense for the first eight hours after delivery and only usually last three to four days.

4. Hearing test

The NHS Newborn Hearing Screening Programme (NHSP) offers all new parents the opportunity to have their baby's hearing screened within the first few weeks of life. Today, many babies will have their hearing tested before leaving the hospital. The tests are simple and painless and only take a few minutes. The new hearing-screening tests use sophisticated technology, can be carried out almost immediately after birth and are much better at identifying a possible hearing impairment than the previous health visitor distraction test done at eight months.

5. An unsettled first night

The first full night that you spend either in the hospital or at home is usually pretty rough. If you have had pain relief such as pethidine or an epidural then your baby may be sleepy for the first day or so and your 'rough night' will be delayed, but it will arrive.

Your baby has been used to being nice and cosy inside the womb for the last nine months. She has been reassured by the noises inside your tummy – your blood rushing around, your heart beating, and noises vibrating from the outside world. When your baby is born and is then just expected to go in a Moses basket or cot to sleep in a dark, quiet house, she can be very unsettled. She will crave the closeness of being held and you will probably find that she will cry each time you try to put her down for any length of time. Swaddling and using rolled-up towels will help her get used to the cot, as they will help her feel cuddled and cosy. This and other sleeping positions are explained in more detail in Chapter 5. In the first couple of days, however, you need to allow her the comfort of being held and sleeping close to you while she gets used to being in the world and all the new challenges that brings. This will reassure her and give her the confidence to be more settled in the long term.

3
Coming home

Coming home is the most wonderful part but also the most terrifying!

After all the build-up and anticipation over your little one's arrival over the past nine months, all parents are looking forward to this moment. However, when you get home and close the door there is inevitably a moment of wondering, 'OK, what do I do now?'

You have this little person whom you created, who is relying on you and is your responsibility for at least the next 18 years. What you do and say, and how you love and care for them, will shape the person they become. It is such a scary thought for all of us, but a perfectly normal one, and experienced by every parent in the world.

There will also most likely be a queue of visitors waiting to pounce on you the moment you get home. Don't be afraid to put them off for a few days while you settle yourself and the baby. Do whatever you feel is right. People will understand.

Labour and birth are exhausting and traumatic for you and your baby. She has been used to being inside you for the last nine months, and being born is a huge change for her, so it's very normal for her to be unsettled for the first week or so, and need to hear or feel you close to her for reassurance.

Try to gracefully accept any help that's offered in the first few weeks. If someone offers to do your ironing for you, or cook a meal and drop it round, then grab the offer with both hands!

Most new mums feel like they have something to prove when they bring the baby home but you don't need to be some kind of superwoman, running around keeping the house spotless and cooking wonderful meals for your partner. This is a sure-fire way to become stressed, which in turn will upset your baby. Let your partner, family and friends help you, especially in the first couple of weeks. This will help you recover from the physical and emotional side of birth, bond with your baby and try to establish a regular daily feeding routine with your baby, whether you decide to breast- or bottle-feed.

Breastfeeding

Breastfeeding is widely publicised as the better option for your newborn for as long as possible rather than giving formula. Mothers are told that it is 'best for your baby', 'helps you to bond quicker and easier' and 'provides your baby with important antibodies to help protect them'.

We all see pictures regularly and reports of women saying how wonderful it is, and so much easier than bottle-feeding. A lot of mums feel very pressured to do it even if they are not keen on the idea. Don't get me wrong, it is a wonderful experience, and does make life easier at times when you are out and about. However, nobody tells you how tough it can be to get to that stage!

I want to be honest about this because so many mums give up on breastfeeding in the first two weeks because they aren't expecting it to be difficult, particularly as it is promoted as the 'easy option'. I have breastfed all three of my children and have worked with hundreds of mothers who have also breastfed, and you have to be very determined to get through the initial two weeks of establishing your milk supply. In saying that, in some cases even the most determined of women will simply not produce enough milk to feed their baby adequately. There are ways that you can try to increase your milk supply, but sometimes it is better for you and your baby to stop and move over to formula feeding, if you are constantly having to top her up with a lot of formula milk – at every feed – particularly if your baby is losing weight. See Chapter 4 for more information.

Breastfeeding should be an enjoyable experience for both you and your baby. It should never be something you dread and wish you didn't have to do. This will only make you resent your baby and in turn affect your bonding with her.

Bottle-feeding

If you have decided to bottle-feed your baby entirely without any form of breastfeeding at all, then that is your choice. A mother should never feel pressured to breastfeed. In my experience of chatting to many mums-to-be, it seems to be something that women feel strongly one way or another. You either want to try it or the thought revolts you. It is a totally personal choice.

A bottle-fed baby will not necessarily sleep through the night faster than a breastfed baby, as some books suggest. It varies from baby to baby. In fact one baby I looked after, Theo, dropped his night feed from the age of five weeks, the earliest I have known a baby to do so, and he was totally breastfed for all day feeds and just had one bottle of formula at 10 p.m.

The biggest advantage to bottle-feeding exclusively is that you can see how much she has taken at each feed, and it is generally easier to get your baby into a routine of taking a certain amount of milk much quicker than with a breastfed baby. As long as you keep her feeding at three-to-four-hourly intervals during the day then she will be able to manage one longer stretch in any 24-hour period – you can guide her towards achieving this at night-time. Don't be tempted to let her sleep past feed times during the day. You will end up regretting it at night-time when she will be determined to make up for it!

All babies, even from newborn, can manage one four-to-six-hour stretch between feeds in a 24-hour period. It is up to you to control when she does that longer stretch, and obviously the ideal time would be when you would like your biggest stretch of sleep. See the feeding schedule discussed in Chapter 4 for more information on how to get started.

Bonding

Bonding is not necessarily something that magically happens when your baby is born. It is usually a growing feeling between the two of you that happens over time. For some mothers this begins to happen as soon as they find out they are pregnant, is strengthened when they feel those first movements and kicks, and is heightened to a point they never imagined possible the first time that they hold their baby. For others, the bonding process won't even begin until their baby is born, and will then be a gradual process over time as their baby begins to smile and develop a personality. You may look at your baby's screwed-up face after birth and not be quite sure what to think! The realisation that you are responsible for this little person is terrifying and, even though you may not get a flood of maternal love immediately, you will definitely learn to love your baby.

Dads in particular may find it difficult to form a bond with a baby before they are born. The initial first few months filled with sleep-deprived nights can also make it difficult to feel much love for this little person who is determined to keep everyone awake. If the baby is being breastfed it is even more difficult for the father to play a big part, as the baby will rely on Mum for feeding, but also for soothing a lot of the time. Many dads can feel very pushed out during the first few months after a baby is born, and not really understand their place and what they can do to help. I always advise the fathers of the babies I look after to just try to be as supportive of Mum as possible. They can help her out by taking on a lot of the household chores so that she can concentrate on the baby, without the worry of mess around her, and cooking a healthy meal so that she can keep her energy stores up. Mothers will really appreciate this type of help – I know I did!

Most fathers don't really get a chance to feel like they are beginning to bond with their child until they are a few months old. This usually coincides with the baby developing a personality – smiling, giggling and cooing. It's wonderful to finally start getting something back from your baby, after what may seem like an endless round of sleep-deprived nights!

There are ways that will encourage and deepen your bond with your baby that both parents can do:

- **Cuddle her frequently**. Skin-to-skin contact particularly in the first few weeks will be a lovely experience for both of you. It's something that Mum and Dad can do.
- **Talk to her constantly**, about anything and everything, even what you are doing as you walk around the house. She will love to hear the sound of both Mum's and Dad's voice, and will learn to recognise both of them very quickly and be soothed by them when she's upset.
- **Watch her as she sleeps for a few minutes every day**. Babies and older children have such a calm, peaceful look about them as they sleep. This is a particularly helpful thing to try if you have had a rough day. She will look so angelic that your bad day fades into the background as you watch her sleep. I still creep in to look at all three of my children as they are sleeping before I go to bed myself, and they are much older now. As I watch them calmly sleeping I can forgive them all the stress they have caused me throughout the day!

The first couple of weeks

There will be so many new things you will experience in the first couple of weeks, and questions you will no doubt be wondering the answers to. I have compiled a list below of some of the common subjects parents think about initially.

Midwives/health visitor

Your midwife will come and visit you at home once you are discharged from hospital. If you live in a busy town or city it is highly likely you will have more than one midwife and will see a different one each time. She will ask you questions when she visits and check your and your baby's health to make sure everyone is happy with the way things are going. Don't be afraid to bombard her with questions. It is much better to ask than struggle on when a simple answer could help make things easier for you. If you are having problems breastfeeding, she will be able to give you details of your local breastfeeding counsellor, who will come out and do a home visit.

She will also do your baby's Guthrie (or heel prick) test on day seven. A few drops of blood are collected and sent away to test for a metabolic disorder called phenylketonuria or PKU, as well as cystic fibrosis and to be screened for some other conditions too. You will be given a leaflet that explains them all in more detail. You will then be discharged from midwife care around day 10, provided all is well with you and the baby.

Your local health visitor will then be given your details and will contact you within a couple of weeks to come and do a home visit. She will introduce herself and give you details of all the local baby clinics where you can go to get your baby weighed and meet other mums.

Cord/tummy peg

This area needs to be wiped gently all around the remaining cord a few times a day as you do your baby's nappy. Use a clean cotton pad and some cool boiled water to clean off any dry blood. Don't use wet wipes, creams or any other antiseptic wipe in this area unless advised by your doctor.

The remaining cord generally falls off between days seven and ten and you will most likely just find it in your baby's nappy as you go to change her. If your baby was overdue then the likelihood is that it may come off earlier, but if it still hasn't fallen off by the time your midwife wants to discharge you around day 10, she will probably give it a helping hand. Once it does fall off, your baby's 'tummy button', as they are widely known, may be a bit weepy and gooey for a couple of days. Clean as directed above at every nappy change, ensuring that you give a really firm wipe now, as any remaining little bits that do not get cleaned off properly can make her tummy button red and sore and may cause an infection.

Fontanelle

This is the soft spot on the top of your baby's head where her skull hasn't yet fused together. Unbeknown to a lot of people there is also a smaller fontanelle towards the back of the baby's head, which is much less noticeable and very hard to find. The main reason your baby is born with these two openings in the skull is to allow her head to mould and fit through the birth canal during labour, something that wouldn't be possible with a totally fused skull. It also allows room for your baby's brain to grow in the first year.

The posterior fontanelle, at the back of her head, generally closes within three months of birth. The anterior fontanelle is on the top of her head and starts to close when babies are around six months, and is usually totally closed by the time they are 18 months. The fontanelle on the top of your baby's head usually appears flat as part of the shape of her head – you may notice it 'pulsing' if your baby doesn't have a lot of hair. This is totally normal and nothing to worry about. It may also bulge slightly when she cries. However, a fontanelle that bulges persistently should be looked at by a doctor as it may indicate increased pressure inside the head. Equally, a significantly sunken fontanelle should also be seen by a doctor, as this generally indicates dehydration.

Sticky eyes

This is very common for babies in the first few weeks and is due to blocked tear ducts. You may find yellow/white mucus in the inner corner of the eye and the lids may be stuck together when she has slept for a while. Clean each eye with cotton pads and cool boiled water, taking care to use a separate piece for each eye. Wipe from the inside corner (closest to the nose), outwards. You could also try squirting a bit of breast milk into her eye if you are breastfeeding. It has amazing healing powers and will more often than not clear up a sticky eye. Squeeze a few drops into the affected eye before each feed over a couple of days. If the mucus is more of a green colour, and the eye looks particularly red, then see your GP as soon as possible as it may mean your baby has an infection that needs treating with antibiotics.

Reflexes

There are some natural reflexes that your doctor will test for – possibly at birth, but certainly at the six-to-eight-week post-natal check up:

- **Rooting reflex**: If you stroke a newborn baby's cheek, she will immediately turn in that direction with her mouth open ready to suck. This helps her locate the breast or bottle, and you can use this reflex to gain her attention and encourage feeding even if she is sleepy. It lasts for three to four months but may persist when they are sleeping.
- **Sucking reflex**: A newborn will suck when the roof of her mouth is touched, e.g., with the nipple or bottle teat. This reflex is present at birth and lasts two to four months, when involuntary sucking takes over.
- **Startle/Moro reflex**: If your baby is startled by a sudden or loud noise, or a feeling of falling, she will extend her legs, arms and fingers, arch her back, draw her head back and then draw the arms back with fists clenched into the chest. This Moro reflex lasts four to six months.
- **Walking or stepping reflex**: This works best after the fourth day. Hold your baby upright on a table or flat surface, under

her arms, standing her up. She should lift one leg and then the other as if walking 'steps'. This reflex is present from birth, and lasts for varying amounts of time, but usually disappears around two months and comes back much later when they are close to learning to walk.

- **Palmar grasp reflex**: When you touch the palm of your baby's hand, her fingers will curl around and cling to your finger (or any other small object you place in her hand). You may also notice that she will curl her feet and toes when they are touched.
- **Babinski's/plantar reflex**: When the sole of a newborn's foot is gently stroked from heel to toe, her toes will flare upwards and the foot turns in. This reflex lasts between six months and two years, after which the toes curl down when the sole is touched.
- **Tonic neck or fencing reflex**: When placed on her back a baby will turn one way with opposite arms and legs extended and flexed – *en garde*!

Baby acne

Infant acne affects around 40 per cent of newborns and usually begins around two to three weeks after birth, and can sometimes last until your baby is around two to four months old. The definite cause is unknown but it is believed that it is the mother's hormones still circulating in the baby's system that stimulate their sweat glands and cause pimples to develop.

Another factor that contributes is that dirt and germs in the air get into the baby's still developing pores and cause the angry rash and white-headed spots.

The acne usually only affects the face and neck, although it can sometimes spread to the top of the torso. This is because the face and neck are the most sensitive parts of your baby's body, so will always be affected first, particularly as they are usually uncovered and subject to the dirt and germs in the air.

Do not be tempted to squeeze the spots or pick them as this can lead to infection. Wash your baby's face with cool boiled water and clean cotton pads – no soap should be used. If the acne is really bad and dries out your baby's skin, then get your GP to take a look; they may prescribe a cream if the spots/rash doesn't seem to be improving.

All three of my children suffered from baby acne. My middle child had it particularly badly and got to the stage where his entire face and head were red raw. As a parent it's horrible to see your child suffering like that, even while you know it's just a stage they have to go through. Other people's comments did not help, and there were lots of times I had to bite my tongue. I ended up taking my baby to the doctor, and, after trying various creams and even a mild steroid cream, the rash gradually got better and disappeared.

Milk from your baby's breasts

This is very normal in a newborn baby (boy or girl), and is due to the influx of hormones your baby receives via the placenta just before they are born. You may notice the nipple leaks a white substance and her breasts may be swollen. Mention it to your midwife or health visitor if you are worried but as long as you don't squeeze it then the swelling should go down on its own and the milk dry up. You may also notice that a baby boy may have swollen testicles and a baby girl swollen genitals and even a discharge coming out. Again, this is usually nothing to worry about but mention it to your GP if you are not happy and need some reassurance.

Jaundice

Jaundice is a common and usually harmless condition in newborn babies that causes yellowing of the skin and the whites of the eyes. Other possible symptoms include dark urine and pale-coloured stools instead of bright yellow or orange. Jaundice is caused by the build up of bilirubin in the blood. Bilirubin is a yellow substance produced when red blood cells are broken down. The liver should filter the bilirubin from the blood and change it into a form that allows it to be passed out from the baby in stools. In newborn babies the bilirubin can build up too fast for the liver to filter it all out, causing jaundice. This can occur for two reasons: firstly because newborn babies have more red blood cells than adults and the red blood cells have a shorter life span, and secondly because the breakdown and removal of bilirubin is slower in newborn babies than in adults as the liver is still developing. The following information is given via the NHS (www.nhs.uk/conditions/jaundice-newborn):

> Jaundice is one of the most common conditions that can affect newborn babies. It is estimated that 6 out of every 10 babies will develop jaundice (this rises to 8 out of 10 in babies born prematurely), although only around 1 in 20 babies has levels of bilirubin in their blood that are high enough to require medical treatment.
>
> Most cases of jaundice in babies do not require treatment as the symptoms normally pass within 10–14 days (although in a minority of cases symptoms can last longer).

Two out of three of my children had jaundice after birth. My daughter's jaundice disappeared within a few days but my son's hung around for a good two weeks, improving on a daily basis.

Mothers are usually advised to ensure their baby is feeding regularly and taking in enough fluids, and not left to go for very long stretches between feeds (over six to eight hours). Subjecting your baby to a daily dose of sunlight is also very effective too, as the light on the skin helps to break down the bilirubin and encourage the jaundice to pass. A daily walk or lying your baby on the carpet or in her basket in the sunshine that is coming through a window or door in the house is also an idea if you don't feel up to going out. If she still remains jaundiced 14 days after birth then her bilirubin levels will be checked again and action taken if needed.

First bath

Most babies cry the first few times they have a bath. Being lowered naked into water without any warning is a real shock to them and the majority will scream the entire time they are in the water. It is amazing how quickly they forget that they have just been floating around in water for the last nine months. The more you bathe them though, the more they will get used to it, and after a few weeks it begins to become a very enjoyable experience for both of you. There are things that you can do to help your baby begin enjoying bath time as quickly as possible:

- **Use a bath aid**. Babies are like slippery little eels in the bath and are more likely to cry if they don't feel supported and safe. A bath aid will help with this and give you more confidence as you won't be worrying about her slipping out of your hands and going under the water. It also gives you your hands free to splash water over her gently and wash her.
- **Have everything ready before you start** – such as nappies, clothes and a nice warm towel to wrap her in once you are ready to get her out.
- **Talk to her and reassure her** the whole time she is in the bath with a calm voice and a smile on your face as you splash little bits of water over her body. If she senses that you are anxious then she will be too. The sound of your calm voice will help her learn that bath time is a nice experience and not something to be scared of!

Baby blues

After the birth of a baby, just over half of all new mums experience the 'baby blues'. In my experience it usually happens between days three and seven post-birth but can take up to two weeks to take effect. Many find that they are very emotional over a few days and seem to cry over the tiniest of things or even nothing at all! You may find it impossible to cheer up no matter how much you try and find this frustrating as you can't understand the cause.

The baby blues are thought to be caused by the hormonal changes in your body after the birth of your baby. For many of us the baby blues tend to coincide with the time that your breast milk comes in. This is usually a stressful time anyway if you are breastfeeding because your breasts will be feeling so painful and engorged that your baby will be possibly finding it more difficult to latch on.

I distinctly remember my husband walking past the nursery on day four after our daughter was born. My milk had come in and latching on was proving very difficult for my baby on a breast that she had previously found soft and accessible. He backtracked and came in immediately as soon as he saw both me and the baby in floods of frustrated tears! For me the baby blues only lasted a day or two with all three of my children, which is the norm.

If after a couple of weeks you are still feeling very overwhelmed and out of control then it is worth checking your feelings against the signs and symptoms of post-natal depression (PND), discussed in Chapter 7 as well as various other illnesses and conditions.

4
Feeding

All three of my children and all of the babies I have worked with have been fed at certain times of the day from the start. Obviously, while you are in hospital this may be more difficult, as well as in the first couple of days while breastfeeding before your milk comes in. However, it is very important to try to establish a regular daily feeding routine as early as possible. This will prevent your baby getting into the habit of snacking during the day, and if you ensure she feeds enough in the daytime hours, you will never have the problem of a baby who wants or needs to feed all night.

Breastfeeding

Getting breastfeeding off to a good start is paramount in making it work for you and your baby. Many health-care professionals and books that you buy will encourage women to breastfeed on demand. When it is your first baby, and you probably don't really have much of an idea what you are doing, this often leads to mothers offering the breast to the baby every time she wakes. Very quickly, they can end up spiralling into a vicious circle of the baby waking, taking half a feed (i.e., one breast), dozing back off to sleep, and then waking and wanting the second breast and the rest of her feed a couple of hours later. This 'snack feeding' during the day will likely lead to the baby also waking a lot at night too, and then expecting the same regular feeding pattern. Thinking she must be hungry as she is typically rooting around and chewing her hands, the breast will be offered again.

After a few weeks of this constant demand feeding the mother is exhausted, possibly has sore, cracked or bleeding nipples from the constant feeding, and the baby continues to be fractious and unsettled. And this is recommended as the correct way to breastfeed!

The breastfeeding guide that I encourage all of my mothers to use is the very same one that I used when breastfeeding my three babies. It gives your body a chance to get used to this new experience gradually. By building up the amount of time your baby spends on the breast in the first few days before your full milk supply comes in, your nipples are less likely to get sore. With your body only producing colostrum for the first few days, the only thing you will achieve by letting her suck constantly on the breast is very sore nipples, and it is so difficult to persevere through the pain of that and carry on with breastfeeding. I believe that this is the main reason why many mothers do not get beyond the first few weeks of breastfeeding their baby.

My plan below will encourage your breasts to produce milk by putting your baby to the breast regularly, but not for too long or too often, which would mean she is effectively sucking on a fairly empty breast, as the amount of colostrum produced is minimal. It is present in small amounts for the first three days to match the size of your baby's stomach. Most babies do not need additional nutrition during this time. Colostrum has a yellow colour and is high in protein and low in fat and sugar.

The protein content is three times higher than the mature milk that comes in afterwards because it is so rich in antibodies being passed from the mother. These antibodies protect your baby and act as a natural laxative, helping your baby pass their first stools, called meconium (see page 47).

Latching on

A good nursing pillow or plenty of cushions to hand are a must when you are breastfeeding. Even though a newborn baby is relatively light, when you have to hold them in a particular position at the breast for a period of time, they can suddenly become very heavy. Once you have positioned yourself comfortably on a chair or bed, you need to find the most comfortable position for you. There are various positions that can be used and lots of images and videos posted on breastfeeding websites to give mothers an idea of how to sit and where to place the baby. Essentially, you and your baby will very quickly find a position that you both prefer. Below is a picture with various examples of positions you can use when feeding one baby.

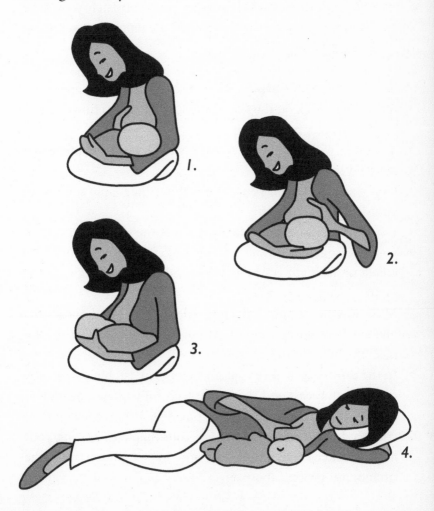

The standard position with which most mothers begin is the 'cradle hold cuddle' (picture 1). Hold her in your arms with her head cradled in your arm of the first breast. You can then use the other hand to help latch her on to the breast.

The 'rugby ball hold' (pictures 2 and 3) is particularly helpful to use with small premature babies, and mothers who have large breasts, to prevent the baby from being buried by the boob! Place a pillow or cushion (I found a V-pillow to be the best) next to you. Place your baby across the cushion so that her legs are facing away from you with her head level with your breast.

By following the steps below every time you latch your baby on to the breast, they will be able to find the nipple and get going much quicker.

- Try to ensure your baby is fully awake before you begin.
- Stroke her cheek on the side that you need her to turn towards the breast. Her rooting reflex will encourage this.
- Tease her with the nipple around her lips until she opens her mouth very wide.
- Cup your breast with your thumb above the nipple and rest of your hand underneath.
- Lift your breast up and when you think the time is right, push your breast into her mouth, trying to get a large amount of the areola underneath your nipple into her mouth along with the nipple. (See picture opposite).
- Make sure her tongue (which should be down underneath the nipple), bottom lip, and chin touch your breast first as you push the breast into her mouth.
- In the early days, before your milk comes in, latching your baby on to your breast and doing the feed isn't usually painful. If you do find that it is painful as your baby begins sucking then you need to break the suction on your nipple by placing your finger between her mouth and your nipple and attempt the latching-on process above again.

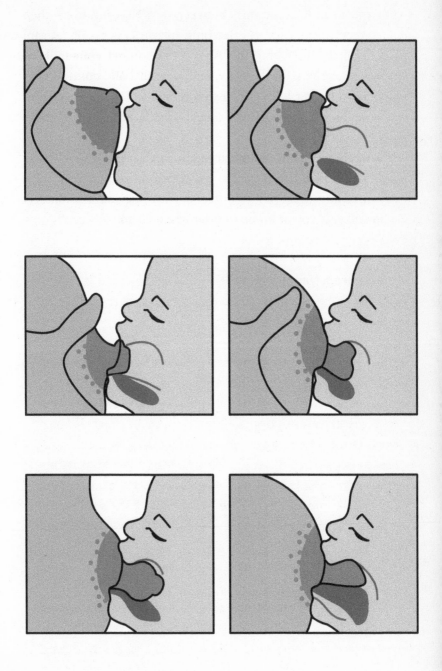

- Once your milk comes in – between days two and five – then it is very normal for the latching-on process to be painful for the first 10–15 seconds. As soon as you get your milk let down then the pain subsides, and as your baby continues to suck it no longer hurts – you should just feel a gentle tugging at your breast as your baby feeds. This is explained in more detail later.

- If you are still having trouble trying to latch your baby on to the breast correctly, then you can ask your midwife for your local breastfeeding counsellor's contact details. They have volunteers who will visit you at home to offer free help and advice.

Initial breastfeeding plan

This can be used from day one to ensure the breasts are stimulated enough but not over-used.

Day 1: *10–15 minutes on the breast at any one time. If she breaks off before this then wind her and reoffer the same breast and allow up to a maximum of 15 minutes. If she is still sucking after 15 minutes then break the suction by placing your finger between her mouth and your nipple, then pull the breast away. Wind her by placing her in one of the positions suggested on page 104. She may not burp that much or even at all in these first few days, as she will not be taking in a lot of fluid at each feed anyway. Offer her the second breast if she is still rooting around after 15 minutes on the first breast, having tried winding her.*

- *Wake your baby every three to four hours in the first couple of days between the hours of 7 a.m. and 10 p.m. This will be crucial in trying to encourage your breasts to begin making milk as quickly as possible. If she is still asleep three hours after her last feed then attempt to wake her up by changing her nappy. This is usually enough to make her want to be put to the breast* immediately afterwards, as newborns do not generally enjoy having their nappy changed!

- If she is still rooting around after you have given her both breasts, then it's a good idea to offer her a clean knuckle or a sterilised dummy to suck on for a bit of comfort. Once she calms down then you can remove the dummy. (See info on dummies on page 29 for more details).

- It is important that you don't let her suck on your nipples for long periods of time in the first few days when you are only producing colostrum. She will have got everything that is available within the 15-minute period anyway, and it is so important that you try to do everything possible to prevent your nipples from becoming sore, or you will find it very difficult to continue breastfeeding.

- Try to have her last feed between 10 and 11 p.m., and then settle your baby and attempt to get some sleep yourself. As mentioned before, a newborn baby is able to manage one four-to-six-hour stretch of sleep without needing to be fed. The most helpful time for this to happen is between 11 p.m. and 4 a.m., so that you are able to get a good stretch of sleep yourself. If she wakes before 3 a.m. then try to settle her back to sleep with a cuddle or stall her with the dummy for a little bit longer.

- Offer her a full feed (both breasts), somewhere between 3 and 4:30 a.m. when she wakes again and then settle her back to sleep. It is hoped that she will then manage to wait until between 7 and 8 a.m. for her next feed. This is more achievable if she has her full breastfeed in the night after 3 a.m. If you have to give it before this time then it's almost certain that you will get a second waking for another feed.

Day 2: Increase your baby's time on each breast to 15–20 minutes. Continue to wake and feed every three to four hours during the day. Leave her to sleep a bit longer between 11 p.m. and 3–4 a.m.

> **Day 3:** *Increase time spent on each breast to a maximum amount of 30 minutes. Until your milk comes in sometime between now and day five she may want to spend a long time on each breast. Once it comes in fully, and she begins to get the mature milk, she will most likely not need to spend as long on the second breast.*

Below is an example of how much an average infant's stomach can take **per feed** on a daily basis. This may help to alleviate some of the perfectly natural worry among breastfeeding mothers about whether their baby is drinking an adequate amount of milk.

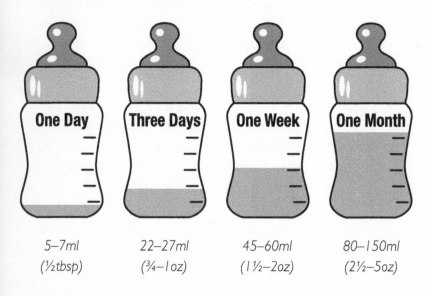

One Day	Three Days	One Week	One Month
5–7ml	22–27ml	45–60ml	80–150ml
(½tbsp)	(¾–1oz)	(1½–2oz)	(2½–5oz)

A bottle-feeding baby may end up drinking more than the above amounts at each feed, or you may find your baby drinks more than this when given expressed milk. As long as your baby is putting on a regular amount of weight then it doesn't matter how much they are drinking at each feed. Sometimes the amounts may even vary from feed to feed or day to day. She will let you know the correct amount for her.

How do I know when my milk has come in?

When your milk comes in your breasts will become gradually harder, and once the milk has completely come in you may even feel lumps in your breasts and under your arms. This is known as **engorgement** and can be very painful.

During the first few days of milk production your breasts will produce as much milk as possible, which means that some milk ducts can become blocked. The amount that you then use that milk supply over the next couple of weeks will determine how much or how little your breasts produce. The engorgement will always be worse just before you are due to feed. If you find that you do have lumps in your breasts or under your arms, you can gently massage them out by pushing them towards the nipple to try to unblock the milk ducts. This can be done at any time, day or night, in between feeds or even while your baby is feeding. Other ways to relieve engorgement are:

- **Placing a warm flannel on the breast** for a couple of minutes before a feed. This should help the milk to flow more freely.
- **Investing in a good comfortable nursing bra**. This will help immensely. A breastfeeding mother should not wear an under-wired bra on a regular daily basis, as it restricts blood flow. (Wearing one for a day or evening out on a special occasion will be fine though.)
- **Using chilled cabbage leaves and ice packs** *after* a feed (not before or during). This can reduce breast pain and discomfort.

When your milk first comes in and your breasts are full, your baby may find it extremely difficult to latch on. She will have got used to a soft breast and nipple, and when your milk comes in and the whole shape of your breast changes she may get very frustrated, as she can't get a proper grip on the nipple to suck. If this happens try manually squeezing some breast milk out of the nipple with your fingers until the areola and nipple become softer. This will allow her to be able to latch on much more easily. As she feeds you will feel continued relief the longer she spends on the breast. If you find yourself producing a massive amount of milk in the early days, then you may need to use a breast pump to express an ounce or so off the breast before offering it to your baby. The excess that you express off can be stockpiled over a 24-hour period and then placed in a freezer bag to freeze, ready for you to defrost and use once you introduce a bottle.

It is very normal for one breast to be better at producing milk than the other, and for one to look visibly smaller (don't worry, nobody else will notice). You will probably find that your baby is always able to finish and empty the smaller breast much quicker than your bigger, fuller breast. This happens to most mums. As long as you always make sure that you use your breasts evenly in terms of switching breasts that you offer first at each feed, then there isn't anything else you can do to improve it. If you put her on the smaller, less productive boob more, then your other breast will begin to make less because it's not being used as much, unless you make sure that you always express any excess milk off after she finishes her feed.

Pain when breastfeeding

As previously mentioned when your mature milk does come in, the latching-on process can suddenly become very painful for a couple of weeks. This surprises first-time mothers as well as mums who may have other children but have never breastfed. This is a very normal phase that the majority of breastfeeding mothers have to go through. However, it doesn't seem to be something that is widely discussed as normal, and I think this is another reason why many mothers give up breastfeeding within the first few weeks.

Mums are often told that breastfeeding is this wonderful experience that is better for you and your baby in many ways and isn't painful at all. You start off well and for the first few days everything runs smoothly: your baby latches on easily, it doesn't hurt at all, she feeds and then goes back to sleep again …

Suddenly it all changes when your mature milk comes in. You now have two giant rocks for breasts. Your baby realises that finally she is going to start getting something for all the effort she is putting in, but can't actually latch on to the breast because it is so full, and a totally different shape. Latching her on becomes very difficult as she gets more and more frustrated with you and the breast. This is tough on you too, because you will be doing your best to help guide her into latching on, but at times you feel like you are going round in circles. She then becomes more and more irate as she gets more and more hungry. She knows it is there in front of her but just can't get on the nipple due to engorgement. All of this also very conveniently coincides with you hitting the baby blues, which is a result of your hormones going into overdrive!

CASE STUDY: My breastfeeding experience

I had a very stressful couple of days with my third baby when my milk came in. She had been breastfeeding beautifully from day one, latching on well and had built up to a regular amount of time on the breast every three to four hours.

On day three my milk came in with a vengeance! I had very full hard breasts and my daughter was finding it more and more difficult to latch on for a feed with each passing hour, as I produced even more milk. I am one of these lucky mums who seem to produce enough to feed an army of babies, which usually I am grateful for, but not in those early days.

*I expressed a couple of ounces off the first breast in order to make it softer and easier for her to latch on to the nipple before each feed. However, after three very scrappy feeds, which took a good 20 minutes of battling to even get her to latch on to the breast, both she and I were very emotional. She was so hungry that with every feed it became more and more difficult to get her to latch on, as she was losing focus. All she knew was that she wanted food, and she wanted it **now**! I was feeling* like a terrible mother, trying to feed my baby but clearly starving her, as she was furious with me. My husband walked past the nursery to find me weeping in the chair, tired, hormonal and feeling defeated, with our screaming hungry daughter in my arms!

Thankfully he was the voice of reason in my emotional state and suggested we offer her a small bottle of expressed milk to satisfy her immediate hunger and calm her down. Admittedly I was very worried about giving her a bottle at a younger age than I had ever done before. However I knew that I was backed into a corner and needed to get a reasonable amount of milk into her for her sake, as she was beside herself with hunger. I also needed to know that she had finally drunk a decent amount of milk so I stopped beating myself up.

I expressed off 3fl oz (90ml) leaving me with a fairly full breast still (I told you I had a massive amount), and my husband offered her the milk from a bottle. She happily drained the full 3fl oz (90ml) and calmed down. 15 minutes later I offered her the breast that I had expressed from and she happily latched straight on and finished her feed. Then I knew it had been the engorgement that was causing the problem, and it all worked out fine in the end. I also had to offer her a bottle of expressed breast milk (EBM) on a few other occasions over the following few days, but I always made sure that I only offered her 2–3fl oz (60–90ml) to quench her initial hunger and then finished off the feed on the breast. (All of my babies have had huge appetites from the start, so this amount worked for her. A smaller amount of EBM may be needed for a baby with a smaller appetite.)

I was very lucky to have a fantastic group of midwives and a health visitor looking after me who were all very practical women, have had their own babies and understood my problems. They all agreed that offering my baby the bottle was totally the right thing to do in that situation and didn't make me feel like I was in the wrong at all. This reassured a hormonal mother who was feeling very guilty.

When your milk comes in the initial point of latching on is usually very painful for the first 10–15 seconds of your baby sucking until you get your milk let down.

The only way I can think to describe the pain is that it feels like somebody is literally sticking lots of needles into your nipple and breast. I used to cope with it by gritting my teeth, swearing under my breath and mentally counting down the 10–15 seconds the pain would take to gradually fade away and pass. It's also worth knowing that you are likely to have to go through this latching-on pain every for those first few weeks. If she decides to drop off the breast for some reason, to wind or rest, then you will have to go through the pain again when you relatch her back on to the same breast. It is very common for babies to 'fall off' and need to be latched on again a few times per breastfeed during the first few weeks of them and you learning the art of feeding. Placing a hand firmly behind her head once she is latched on can help prevent her falling off as much, which is definitely something you will be trying to avoid because you know what sensation to expect when you latch her on again.

The bad news is that nobody warns you that this latching-on pain is normal over a short period of time and does get better. Mothers are always told that if it hurts as their baby is feeding then they must have them latched on incorrectly. This makes them stop, break the baby off and try to latch them on again. When it still hurts over and over again each time they try to latch their baby on, they think they are doing something wrong, as nobody told them that a short period of pain is normal.

The good news is that you are doing it correctly as long as the pain subsides within the first 10–15 seconds as described. You will notice that the pain gradually becomes less and less and then fades away as your milk let down happens.

Some women feel a let down physically in their breast, rather like pins and needles that passes from the top of your breast down towards your nipple. As this happens the latching-on pain fades away at the same time.

Other women will not feel any physical symptoms of a let down, but will be aware of it by the fact that the latching pain has faded, and their baby is now gulping the milk that has come down.

When your baby first latches on, the full milk flow will not be there immediately. She needs to encourage and stimulate your breast to 'let down' this milk with her sucking. The more relaxed and comfortable you are the more easily this will happen. It is quite common for a mother to get a let down from both breasts at the same time, so it is always a good idea to wear a breast pad inside your bra on the opposite breast, to catch any leakage. There are products that can be bought to put inside your bra to catch and store any breast milk that leaks, so that none is wasted – you will very quickly develop the attitude that all breast milk is precious! Breast pads are always worth wearing when you go out and about too. Let downs can occur anywhere at any time – you don't necessarily need to have your baby with you or be about to breastfeed. I had a few embarrassing moments in the middle of the supermarket, and while out and about due to random let downs. Wet patches on your top are really not a great look in public places!

If the latching-on pain doesn't begin to fade after 10–15 seconds, or you get pain midway through a feed, then it's more likely that your baby's position at the breast isn't quite right, and you need to break her suction and try the latching-on process again. Contact your local breastfeeding counsellor if you are still having problems latching your baby on.

This latching-on pain only tends to last for between two and four weeks, after which it subsides and the hard work of getting breastfeeding established begins to feel worth it! Give yourself a big pat on the back and congratulate yourself for all your patience and perseverance. Breastfeeding should feel much easier from now on, and all the benefits begin to become apparent, and make the whole experience much more enjoyable!

What is a 'full breastfeed?'
The breast produces two types of milk as you feed your baby – one that follows on from the other.

Fore milk is the milk your baby gets when they first latch on to the breast. It is thin and watery in consistency with a light blue tinge in colour, and is there to satisfy your baby's thirst.

The milk that follows on from the fore milk is called the **hind milk**. It is a thicker consistency, similar in texture to cream, and has a high concentration of fat. This part of the milk feed fills your baby up, helping her to feel satisfied and gain weight on a regular basis. It is very important that a baby is encouraged to spend long enough on the breast to actually reach this satisfying milk. It will vary from baby to baby as to how long it takes them to reach the hind milk. It will very much depend on the speed at which your baby feeds and how plentiful your milk supply is.

A baby with a very strong suck, who drinks very fast, gulping the milk down initially, can reach the hind milk within five to ten minutes if the mother has lots of milk. A more controlled feeder who takes their time on a mother who has a lower supply of milk, will more likely take 10–15 minutes to reach the hind milk. It's wise to have a digital clock nearby when you feed so that you can keep track of how long your baby has been on the first breast in particular. You will then know when to move her on to the second breast.

There are two ways that you can check if your baby has reached the important hind milk. The first is by watching the way she feeds. When she first latches on to the breast and is drinking the fore milk, she will be sucking almost continuously without pausing and just swallow as she goes.

Once she reaches the hind milk her sucking will calm down a lot. You will notice her doing a few sucks and then pausing for five seconds or so and then sucking again. As the hind milk is thicker, she needs to take her time a bit more and not guzzle it down, or she will be more likely to vomit. If you notice her pause for longer than 10 seconds then you can give her cheek a little stroke or move your nipple slightly while it still remains in her mouth, to stimulate her to begin sucking again.

The second way to check if your baby has reached the hind milk is when you take her off the breast to wind. Gently squeeze your nipple and look at the milk that comes out. As described above, fore milk will most likely squirt out very easily and be very watery. The hind milk will look much thicker and may just trickle out as you squeeze the nipple.

Once your milk comes in it is important that you encourage your baby to take a full feed at the times suggested to enable her to reach the important fatty hind milk, and gain a regular amount of weight.

She should be encouraged to stay on the first breast for between 20 and 30 minutes. If she wants to stop after 10–15 minutes on the breast as she has wind, then make sure that you put her back on the same breast to finish off. She will start off exactly where she left off, and continue making her way to the hind milk as long as you continue on the same breast within a short space of time. Let her continue on the first breast for a maximum of 30 minutes (although if you are a few minutes over this it doesn't matter). Even a very slow feeder should have got a good amount of hind milk by this time, and allowing her to continue longer than around 30 minutes will make you more likely to get sore nipples. Break the suction by placing your finger in the corner of her mouth and gently pulling your nipple away.

At this point give your nipple a squeeze and check that it is hind milk that comes out to reassure yourself that she has been sucking and feeding effectively, and not just using the breast for comfort. Most babies close their eyes and look asleep as soon as they begin breastfeeding. They are enjoying the comfort and experience of being so close to Mummy, and closing their eyes is a way of showing this. In reality, if you were to break the suction and take the breast away they would likely open their eyes immediately and root around for the breast again. If you watch her carefully as she feeds and are aware that she is still sucking regularly, even with pauses in between, and hasn't just fallen asleep at the breast, then she should be drawing enough milk from you to keep her satisfied. If she does pause for too long, and stroking her cheek or moving your nipple slightly in her mouth doesn't encourage her to suck again, then you will need to break the suction and take the breast away. Sit her up and wind her, as this may be why she has come to a halt.

Other ways to encourage her to wake up and finish her feed are:

- **A nappy change** – or at least the threat of one! Undress her as if you are going to change her. This generally wakes a baby up enough for them to look for the breast again.
- **Gently tickling** her feet and down the sides of her body. This will rouse her and wake her up.
- **Taking off some layers of clothing**. Having close contact with Mum can make a baby very warm anyway, so try to take some clothes off when it is time for a feed so she doesn't get too hot. She will be more likely to fall asleep at the breast if she's very warm.

Once she has had 20–30 minutes on the first breast you need to encourage her to take something at least from the second breast. Generally most babies only have 5–10 minutes on the second breast if they have taken a decent enough amount of milk from the first breast. If you find that your baby is spending longer than 10 minutes on the second breast regularly, then you need to increase the amount of time she is spending on the first breast in order that she gets more of the hind milk to fill her up.

Generally 30 minutes is enough and your breast should feel much softer and almost empty after that period of time. However, if your baby was very sleepy during the whole feed then she may have not been sucking effectively enough to draw the milk out. This is common, particularly in the first few weeks when a newborn falls asleep constantly. Use the methods described previously to try to get an effective feed into her.

Once your baby has had enough milk from the second breast then she will have had a full feed. It is wise to use a hair bobble, bracelet or watch to put on the wrist of the same side breast that you finished the feed on if she did take both breasts. You should always start a breastfeed on the breast that you finished on at the last feed. This will ensure that each breast is emptied at every other feed, and you are using them equally. By putting something on your wrist it will remind you which breast you need to begin on. Sleep deprivation causes you to be very forgetful and even trying to remember something as simple as which breast you last fed on is near impossible. In the early days your breasts will be producing so much milk and be so full that you won't even be able to tell by feeling the weight of them, as they will reproduce and fill up again very quickly after the last feed.

If your baby point blank refuses the second breast after having 30 minutes on the first one, and you have tried winding and all of the methods to attempt to wake her, then don't worry. It may be that she had such a good amount of hind milk from the first breast that she doesn't feel hungry enough to take the second breast, even after a short break. If that's the case then I would advise that you express some milk off the second breast using your breast pump.

This is important for two reasons:

- You will be in a lot of pain if you don't, particularly in the early days when your breasts may be very engorged and full of milk.
- It will encourage your breasts to keep producing a good supply of milk.

Just because your baby only took one breast at a particular feed that doesn't mean that she won't want both breasts next time. Milk is produced on a supply-and-demand basis. If the milk from the second breast isn't used, and doesn't get expressed off, it gives the message to your body not to make that much milk as it isn't needed.

Expressing will encourage your breasts to continue making as much milk as possible, which is particularly important for when your baby goes through growth spurts and suddenly decides that she does want that extra milk. If you have been expressing after a feed, it will already be there for her to have. If you haven't been expressing then it will take your body a day or two to catch up with the extra demand, which means you will likely have a fractious baby in the meantime wanting more milk than she is actually getting!

Any excess milk pumped off can be placed in a breast milk freezer bag (see page 25) and put in the freezer to use at a later date. Milk produced at separate feed times over a 24-hour period can be mixed together and placed in a single freezer bag. The only thing you need to remember is not to mix fresh, warm, recently expressed breast milk with the cold milk already stored in the fridge. You can store them in two separate containers in the fridge and wait until they are both at the same temperature before you mix them together.

Below is a table of the recommended breast milk storage guidelines at room temperature, in the fridge and in the freezer.

Place of storage	Temperature	Maximum storage time
In a room	25°C/77°F	Six–eight hours
Insulated thermal bag with ice packs		Up to 24 hours
Refrigerator (in the body of fridge, NOT the door)	4°C/39°F	Five days max
Freezer compartment inside a refrigerator	-15°C/5°F	Two weeks
Combined fridge and freezer with separate doors	-18°C/0.4°F	Three to six months
Chest or upright manual defrost deep freezer	-20°C /-4°F	Six to twelve months

Recommended breastfeeding times

In the places where I have written two times next to each other then the first time stated is the earliest time you should ideally start to feed, and the second time stated is the latest time the feed should begin. This will enable you to try to stay on track with feeds in order to ensure you get enough milk into your baby on a daily basis and one feed time doesn't drift into the next one.

The feeding times that I suggest as a guide to all my breastfeeding mums are exactly the same as the times for a mother who is formula-feeding her baby from a bottle. Please see below:

7/7:30 a.m. Full feed

10:30/11 a.m. Full feed

2:15/2:30 p.m. Full feed

4:30/5 p.m. One breast

6/6:15 p.m. finish breast used in 5 p.m. feed first, then offer second breast

10:15/10:45 Full feed (eventually leading to bottle of EBM or formula)

3/4:30 a.m. Full feed (possibly changing to bottle of EBM to drop the night feed more easily)

A typical breastfeeding day

I breastfed all three of my children from the day they were born and did all of the things that I am advising you and many mothers before. We all have good days and bad days where we end up slightly out of sync for one reason or another, but on the whole I and all the mothers I have worked alongside have found having these guidelines a huge help. Having the times to work with gave me something to focus on. It also meant that I could plan certain things because I knew roughly when I would be feeding, rather than demand feeding my baby every hour or so which is a common situation for a lot of mums.

Below is a summary and example of what may be a typical day to give you an idea of how to use your breasts evenly as described:

7:15 a.m.   First breast (R) 28 minutes
Second breast (L) 7 minutes. Expressed afterwards

10:30 a.m.   First breast (L) 30 minutes
Second breast (R) 5 minutes. Expressed afterwards

2:15 p.m.   First breast (R) 25 minutes
Second breast (L) 3 minutes. Expressed afterwards

5 p.m.   One breast (L) 25 minutes

6 p.m.   Finished (L) breast 8 minutes
Second breast (R) 20 minutes

10:30 p.m.   First breast (R) 27 minutes
Second breast (L) 6 minutes

3:30 a.m.   First breast (L) 25 minutes
Second breast (R) 4 minutes

The next morning ...

7:30 a.m.   First breast (R) 20 minutes
Second breast (L) 10 minutes

The above is an example of a very good day of feeding to help you understand how and when to give each breast and what constitutes a full feed. In making sure your baby is encouraged to reach the important hind milk at each feed by spending long enough on the first breast, you will never reach the scenario of having a baby up all night feeding.

The only feed that doesn't need to be a full feed is the 5 p.m. one. This feed is given initially in the first few weeks because a very young baby struggles to do the 2:30–6 p.m. stretch, more so if they are breastfed. I have found that if you offer one breast and then let the milk settle before bathing her and offering the rest of the feed, she should then be ready to settle down to sleep for the remainder of the evening until the next feed. This is the only feed where your baby will spend longer on the second breast at 6 p.m. because the first breast will have already been almost emptied one hour earlier.

A lot of midwives and health professionals advise mothers to breastfeed on demand. As a new mum on a huge learning curve every day, it is very difficult to gauge what this means. When a newborn baby wakes she will immediately start eating her hands and anything that comes into contact with her mouth in search of food. It is very easy to slip into the habit of feeding her immediately while she is still sleepy. She will likely then take a quick 10-minute snack feed and fall back to sleep.

The problem is that she will have only taken a quick drink of the fore milk. A 10-minute feed is not long enough to have had a sufficient amount of hind milk to sustain her for a few hours, therefore she will wake again after another hour or two, and the same cycle happens again. Thus beginning a vicious circle of snack feeding. As she hasn't got enough of the fatty hind milk into her during the day, this snack feeding will continue all through the night too.

After a few weeks of this the mother becomes exhausted, the baby is fractious and nobody is enjoying the experience. Being advised to do this demand feeding is why I believe a lot of mothers give up breastfeeding within the first few weeks. It is simply too tiring, time consuming and apparently endless as the baby seems no less settled from the constant feeding. Once a mother begins to understand the differences between the two milks, it makes it more reasonable to persevere with encouraging her to wait a bit longer between feeds, in order to build up a better appetite and take a more substantial feed.

Your diet while breastfeeding

The crucial thing to remember is that everything you eat, drink or take is likely to go into your breast milk and possibly affect your baby in various ways. Therefore it is vital that you try to eat a balanced diet, drink plenty of fluids, and make sure your doctor is aware that you are breastfeeding if he needs to prescribe you any medication.

Breastfeeding tends to make most mothers feel very hungry and thirsty anyway, so that alone should encourage you to eat and drink enough. Eating little and often is the key to a good milk supply. Your body will be using extra calories to produce the milk, so you may even find yourself losing weight despite being ravenous and eating like a horse!

CASE STUDY: Breastfeeding and losing weight

There was a standing joke between me and Sally – a mother of twins, who was solely breastfeeding them. Every time I arrived at the house and she opened the door I would say, 'For goodness' sake, woman, will you just eat something,' and she would laugh and say, 'Lisa, I literally don't stop eating!' She was stick thin by the time the girls were eight weeks old because the demands of breastfeeding were burning off so many calories! After spending a few days with her establishing the girls' routine I knew that she definitely was eating vast amounts of food just to keep up her milk and energy supplies. After I had all three of my babies I would find I was getting on the scales every morning to weigh myself and was losing 3–4lb (1.3–1.8kg) a day, despite eating whenever I could as I was permanently hungry from breastfeeding.

Taking in enough fluid is also essential. The best thing to drink is still water, as this will be the best way to replace the fluid that you are feeding to your baby. Flavoured water is fine too if you can't bear the taste of plain old tap or bottled water. I personally found that putting bottles of water in the fridge overnight made them much more refreshing to drink the following day. I also found it much easier to just grab another bottle of water from the fridge and have it as one of my essential items needed when it was time to sit down and breastfeed. I used to aim to drink between 500ml and 1 litre of water every time I breastfed and then drink extra fluid in between feeds if I was thirsty.

Tea, coffee and carbonated drinks are fine in moderation, but be aware of how much caffeine you are taking in, as this can affect your baby in the same way it affects you, making them more alert and wakeful. It is also one of the triggers linked to colicky babies.

The balance of fruit, vegetables and other things you eat is important too. Certain foods you eat can change your baby's bowel habits and also affect how windy she is. If spicy foods are not a regular part of your diet, they can make your baby unsettled a day or so later. I would advise everything in moderation, and suggest you watch your baby for any adverse reaction to the foods you eat, particularly the unusual ones.

Dairy intolerances are very common in babies, and can cause colic or even reflux in your baby. (See colic/reflux section on page 108 for more information, and for what to do if you feel this may be causing a problem.)

A breastfeeding mother needs to ensure she is getting enough fruit, vegetables and fibre in her diet to help her baby to open her bowels regularly. It is very easy to forget that what you eat will also affect your baby's digestive system. If you suffer from constipation then it is likely your baby's bowel movements may not be as regular as some of your friends' babies. I found orange juice was a great thing to drink when breastfeeding if I noticed that my baby hadn't had a bowel movement for a few days. She would clear her bowels out 24–48 hours later, and it has also worked for many other mums' babies. It's a good idea to drink it in moderation though as, if you are having a glass or two every day, then you may get a few too many unwanted nappies to change! One of my breastfeeding mums discovered this as she used to drink a lot of juice, and as soon as she limited her intake her baby's bowel movements calmed down.

Vitamins and supplements help ensure you are getting all of the nutrients you and your baby need to stay healthy while breastfeeding. These can be bought in your local supermarket or pharmacy, and there are pills specifically aimed at breastfeeding mothers. You should find them on the baby aisle or the medicine aisle.

Top-ups

Your breasts will work on a supply-and-demand basis, so the more milk you use the more they will continue to produce.

However, it is possible in some circumstances that mothers experience this initial engorgement but are then never able to produce enough milk, long term, to satisfy their baby with breast milk alone. If you are worried that this may be happening then you can top-up your baby with any expressed milk you are able to pump off in the early days when your milk supply is more plentiful. If formula top-ups need to be introduced because your baby doesn't seem satisfied after each feed, then initially offer them after the 6 p.m. and 10:30 p.m. breastfeeds. This will ensure that your baby definitely gets a full feed at the end of the day when it's more likely your supply will be lower. This will also enable her to have a more settled sleep at night and prevent her having to snack all night to try to make up for what she may be missing out on during the day.

Any amount of breast milk that you can give your baby will benefit her so always offer her a full breastfeed and any expressed milk you have first, before any formula top-ups.

There are also certain products that are thought to boost milk production if you are worried that you are not producing enough. Herbal remedies as well as medicine prescribed from a doctor can sometimes help. Talk to your midwife, doctor or health visitor for the best current recommendation to boost your milk supply.

Stress will have a big impact on your milk supply. It can particularly affect your let down of milk, so try to be as relaxed as possible when it's time for a feed or you need to express. Reading a book/magazine (once you get more experienced at breastfeeding), or just watching your favourite TV programme can help put you in a more relaxed mood.

Breastfeeding twins

If you have twins I would advise sticking to the same feed times as I have suggested for a single baby. A full feed for twins is different however.

Each baby should be offered one breast each and I wouldn't recommend swapping for the duration of any one feed. I would advise allowing each baby a maximum of 45 minutes as their total feeding time on the breast. Obviously you will have winding breaks within the duration of the feed. It is very unlikely either twin will feed for 45 minutes solid without stopping. Build up to this duration gradually though, just as suggested for a single baby, from when you are only producing colostrum to when your mature milk arrives.

You are bound to find that your babies drink at different speeds, and one may always like to spend longer on the breast than the other. Because of this it is very important that you alternate which breast each twin has at every feed. If twin one had the right breast at the 7 a.m. feed, then give her the left breast at the 10:30 a.m. feed then the right at 2:30 p.m., and so on. You don't want to end up feeling lopsided by having one breast producing more than the other as you always put the hungrier twin on the same side.

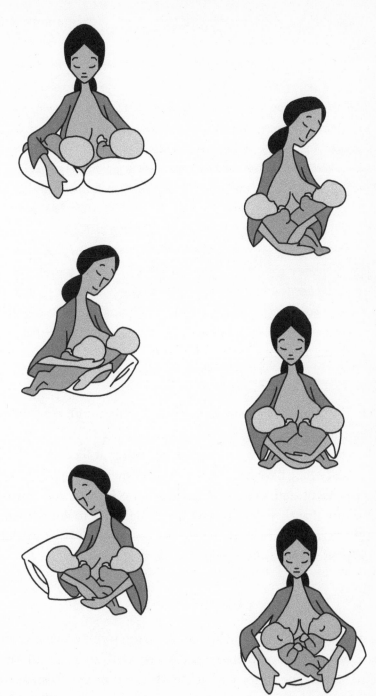

> **Tip**
>
> In the first few weeks always do the scheduled day feeds at the same time with both babies. Don't be tempted to let one baby sleep past the feed time in the hope that you will be able to finish feeding the first twin before the second wakes. You can almost guarantee it will never work out like that. In my experience I have found that twins tend to have a sixth sense when the other one is being fed. You never end up making it to the end of the feed, and will actually make more work for yourself in messing around with nappy changes for number one, while number two is wondering why she has had to stop mid feed.
>
> Always wake your other baby once the first twin wakes and needs feeding in the night and feed them together. Once they are over six weeks old and you start the action plan to drop the night feed, that is when I would suggest leaving the twin that usually sleeps for longer to continue sleeping. You do generally find that you will have one baby who drops the night feed earlier than the other one.

As they get older your babies will become more efficient at feeding anyway, and begin to drink their full feed in a faster time. This is normal – they will have just got better at feeding with all the practice they have had, and, as long as they are happily going between feeds and gaining weight each week, then you can be pretty sure that they must be getting enough milk to satisfy them. There are some pictures of the various positions on page 91 that mothers use to breastfeed their twins at the same time.

Bottle-feeding

Most infant formula can be bought in carton form, which is ready made, as well as in powdered form, which needs to be mixed with boiled water. The cartons are great for convenience, particularly when out and about, but are the most expensive option. The powdered formula is the cheapest way to feed your baby when bottle-feeding and you will need to make up the feeds every day. There will always be instructions on the tub giving you guidance on how to make the feed and a rough estimate of how much your baby should be taking at each feed at various ages. This is not set in stone though, so be guided by your baby as to how much is enough. If she is draining each bottle and looking for more milk long before the next feed time, then you need to increase the amount you are giving her at each feed by 1fl oz (30ml). If a few weeks later she is draining the new amount, then increase her day feeds by another ounce (30ml). Be aware though that some babies who finish their feeds very quickly may look for more milk again straight after winding. Try to make her wait 15–30 minutes if she has taken the feed fast, to make sure she is genuinely hungry and not just wanting to suck for comfort. When milk is drunk very quickly it takes time for it to work its way down to a baby's tummy, and for her to realise that she is not actually hungry any more. If she is still rooting around after the waiting period then you can offer more milk.

The only feed that you do not need to keep increasing is the 3/4 a.m. night feed. That bottle should never go over a maximum of 4fl oz (120ml), otherwise it will be more difficult to convince her to drop that feed. If she is getting enough milk during her day feeds, she will never look for more than 4fl oz (120ml) during the night feed anyway.

Overleaf I have listed the feed times that you can use as a guide and implement from the day you come home from hospital and get settled in at home. Changes to these feed times are discussed later on in this chapter on how and when to do this.

Where I have written two times next to each other, the first time stated is the earliest you should try to begin the feed and the second time is the latest time to start to ensure you don't begin to feed too late and put your baby off the next feed.

Recommended bottle-feeding times
7/7:30 a.m.

10:30/11 a.m. Initially may be 10:30 but aim to stretch to a regular time of 11 a.m. as soon as baby can wait the extra time.

2:15/2:45 p.m.

5 p.m. Small top-up of half a feed if needed. Not always essential with formula-fed babies and should be phased out and dropped by around eight weeks

6/6:15 p.m.

10:15/10:45 p.m.

3/4:30 a.m. Let baby wake naturally to ask for this

Try to ensure that your baby takes a full bottle-feed of their current regular amount at each of the above times, and not just a little snack feed. This will help her 'go the distance' between feeds, and not need to look for milk before the next scheduled feed time. Some babies like to be winded halfway through a feed, while others will happily drain the entire bottle and just require winding at the end. Be guided by your baby. You will know when she needs winding, as she will just begin to get very wriggly and fuss as she is drinking the bottle. This is a good indication that you need to stop feeding and check for wind. After a burp or two you will probably find she will then happily drink some more milk, although some babies like a little break before they will finish the bottle.

You can take up to an hour to complete the feed from the time that you start feeding your baby. After an hour, any remaining milk needs to be thrown away. This is because the formula can be a breeding ground for bacteria to grow once it is mixed with your baby's saliva, and she could be more likely to pick up stomach bugs. It is also helpful to make yourself stick within this time frame to prevent feeds running into each other.

If your baby has had what you feel is a full feed at the guide time and is showing signs of being hungry, then I would suggest you try settling her by offering the dummy. Babies naturally 'root around' every time they wake up in the first few weeks. This is normal and doesn't always mean that you have to feed her. By using a dummy to satisfy her urge to suck, it's very likely that you will be able to resettle her back to sleep, or calm her down enough to realise that she isn't frantically hungry, and will be able to wait a bit longer until the next feed time. See the section on dummies on page 29 for more details.

If she really won't settle with the dummy, is still rooting around for milk and crying despite your best efforts to 'stall' and still has more than an hour to wait until the next scheduled feed time, then it is okay to give her a little more. Try to get away with as little milk as possible, and treat this extra feed as a top-up. Don't be tempted to allow her to have a big milk feed at this time, as you still need to offer a full feed at the next time that she would be due anyway. This way you are always aiming to get her back on track with the set feed times, but you are also satisfying her extra milk need. She will then learn to cope without these top-ups if you always ensure she gets a full feed regularly throughout the daytime.

With a newborn baby I would advise that you start off by using a number 1 slow-flow teat on her bottles. As she gets older you can move her through the numbered teats to faster-flowing teats – numbers 3 or 4 being the fastest, depending on what brand of bottles you are using. Again, be guided by your baby when she is ready to move up to a faster-flowing teat. If she is taking fairly small amounts at each feed, then it is worth trying her on a faster-flowing teat just to see if it helps her pick up on the amount of milk that she drinks. I would advise this particularly if she is not putting on a vast amount of weight, even if she has been happily going from one feed to the next.

Another indicator that it is time to move up to the next-sized teat is when a baby has been regularly drinking a certain amount at each feed, but then begins to have a period over a few days or more where she doesn't finish her milk, or perhaps only takes half of it. If she is otherwise well in herself and not showing any signs of illness, then the reason for this apparent 'loss of appetite' could be due to the bottle teat. If a baby finds that it is quite hard work to extract the milk from the bottle, then she can become bored and give up trying after a while, particularly if you had heated the milk and it has gone cold by this point. She will take the initial amount from the bottle, as she is hungry and the milk is warm, but once winded and when the milk has lost its temperature, she may lose interest and find it all too much like hard work. As she has satisfied her initial hunger, her enthusiasm will dip and she may not want to finish the milk.

If you get to this stage it is important that you don't resort to snack feeding your baby. When she is taking less milk at each feed suddenly, she may start to struggle to wait for the next feed at the usual time. Snack feeding can lead to a whole host of other problems like excess wind and colic, so you really don't want to go down that route.

If you notice this habit of reduced feeding over a few days and your baby obviously needs to take more as she is struggling to wait between feeds, then I would advise that you move her on to the next-sized teat as soon as possible.

Some teats have a certain recommended age on their packaging. Ignore this: it is a guide only and not set in stone. Be guided by *your* baby. They all suck differently and some have a stronger suck than others. Most newborns move on to the level 2 teat within the first month anyway, although it is a good idea to stick to a level 1 teat purely for the night feed, even if you change to a faster-flowing teat during the day. This will discourage her from taking a big feed at night, particularly as she will be less alert. This, in turn, will make it easier to drop the night feed. Persevere with the faster-flowing teat over a few days – it's normal for her to splutter a bit the first few times you use the faster-flow teat, as she needs to adapt her sucking to the new milk flow. She will soon get the idea.

How to sterilise and make feeds

All bottles, teats and feeding equipment need to be washed thoroughly then placed in a steriliser. See directions below:

- Fill a bowl with hot, soapy water using washing-up liquid.
- Soak the bottles, then wash thoroughly using your bottlebrush. Ensure you clean all milk deposits out of the teats in particular.
- Rinse everything with hot or cold water to wash off all the bubbles.
- Place the bottles in the steriliser and switch on with the correct amount of water added according to manufacturer instructions.

Bottles can be prepared in two ways:

1: Mix the boiled water and formula together in advance and store 24 hours' worth of feeds in the fridge. When needed, the already prepared milk can be heated slightly to take the fridge chill off the milk and then given to your baby at room temperature.

2: Make the bottles with the correct amount of water in for the feed 24 hours in advance. Store in the fridge. When needed, heat the water so that it is warm and then add the correct amount of scoops of formula. Shake and serve! (It is important that you heat the water to a fairly warm temperature, otherwise the scoops of formula will not dissolve properly and you will end up with lumps that block the teat.)

Below are directions on how to make a formula feed once your bottles have already been sterilised. You will also find similar instructions on the side of any tub of formula:

- Wash your hands with anti-bacterial soap.
- Empty out the kettle and fill with fresh water. Boil once. Babies' feed should always be made with fresh once-boiled water. If you are not sure if the water has been pre-boiled at any time (maybe by another household member), then you must throw it away and boil with fresh water. When you boil water repeatedly it changes the mineral content of the H_2O, so it's very important that you stick to this simple rule. Do not use water that has been softened using a water softener to make up your baby's feeds either.
- While the kettle is boiling, spray the work surface where you plan to make the feeds with bleach. Wipe dry with a fresh piece of kitchen roll. It is not a good idea to use sponges or cloths to clean, or tea towels to dry the surface, as these items are a very high breeding ground for germs. Babies are very sensitive to picking up tummy bugs, so high levels of hygiene are essential.
- Remove the sterilised bottles from your steriliser and line them up on the worktop with the measuring numbers facing you.
- Fill the bottles to the required amount of ounces/millilitres that your baby is currently taking with cool boiled water.
- If you would like to make the bottles up completely in advance for the next 24 hours, then now is the time to put in the scoops of formula. The basic rule to remember is to use one scoop per 1fl oz (30ml) of water. The water that you add the scoops to needs to be cooled but still warm, otherwise the formula will not dissolve properly.
- Shake thoroughly with the teat and lid on. Use one teat and lid to shake and mix the milk by moving it on to the next bottle as you go. Once all of the bottles have had the formula and water mixed together, put a sterilised teat and lid on each of them – one that doesn't have milk residue in from making up the feeds. Wash and re-sterilise the final teat that was used for shaking and mixing the formula.

- You can then store the pre-prepared feeds in a fridge for a maximum of 24 hours. Ensure they are stored in the body of the fridge and not the door.
- Always make up one extra bottle of boiled water regardless of which method you use to make up your feeds, just in case you need it at some point. This could be due to a feed being spilled or dropped (which happens more than you would think), or the baby needing some extra milk, particularly during growth spurts.
- If you would rather make up the feeds as you need them, then the teats and lids can be put on the bottles of the boiled water and placed in the body of the fridge until needed.
- Take the bottle of water out of the fridge when your baby is due for a feed and heat it so that the water is very warm but not hot. Use one of the methods described on page 34 to heat the water. It is important that the water is fairly warm otherwise the formula will not dissolve properly. SHAKE.
- Check the temperature of the milk by pouring a little on the inside of your wrist. This is one of the most sensitive parts of an adult's body.
- If temperature is okay, then you can begin to feed your baby.

Feeding your baby

- Make sure you have everything you need close by before you start, including a bib and muslin plus spares, just in case your baby vomits.
- Sit yourself in a comfortable chair and position your baby in the crook of your arm sitting slightly upright. If she is completely flat as you feed her she is more likely to choke and vomit the feed back up again. Alternatively if a baby is sat completely upright it will be very uncomfortable for her as she drinks the milk. Aim for somewhere between the two.
- Tease her mouth with the teat of the bottle as she roots around looking for her milk. Allow her to draw the teat into her mouth

herself rather than you just pushing it straight in, as she will be less likely to gag on it if she does it herself.

- Once you put the bottle in her mouth ensure that the teat is completely full of milk all the time to prevent your baby taking in any excess air. The only point during the feed where the teat won't be full of milk will be as she drains the last of the feed and finishes the bottle.
- Be guided by your baby in terms of winding. If she begins to squirm and wriggle around as she's drinking and fuss on the teat, it is a big indicator that she needs to burp.
- Stop feeding and sit her up or put her over your shoulder to help her get the wind out. (See the pictures and more details on winding at the end of the chapter, page 104.)
- You can then continue the feed and she will hopefully finish the bottle. Some babies prefer a 10–20-minute break before finishing the remaining milk. Others will quite happily drain the entire bottle before they need winding at the end of the feed.

Bottle-feeding twins

The bottle-feeding times for twins are the same as I have listed for a single baby. I always recommend feeding twins at the same time, rather than doing them one after the other as some suggest. I have tended to find it easier that way. If you try consecutive feeds and the first baby takes longer to feed than you expect due to wind, nappy changes, etc., you will delay your other baby's feed even longer. If you end up doing this regularly during the day, and have a few longer stretches between feeds, then she will be much less likely to be able to manage a longer stretch at night-time. As your babies get older and understand and recognise the bottle they are unlikely to be prepared to wait while you feed their sibling.

You will very quickly learn how to bottle-feed and wind two babies at the same time. Practice makes perfect: the more times you do it, the better you will get at it. There is no right or wrong way to do it, but you need to find a method that suits you and your babies.

Bouncy chairs are a big help in feeding twins. If you have bought the type that has an adjustable reclining position then you will be able to alter it to suit the best feeding position for each of your babies.

The other way to feed them would be to prop yourself up on a very large sofa or bed with lots of soft pillows and cushions to keep everybody propped in a comfortable position, particularly if you are doing the feed on your own. There are cushions and pillows that can be bought for feeding twins specifically, but these are fairly expensive, and I have always found that a V-pillow (a much cheaper option), works just as well, coupled with a range of other standard bed pillows or sofa scatter cushions.

When each baby needs winding, you can lift one over each shoulder and pat their backs – two hands for two babies! It only becomes more difficult to wind them together as they begin piling on the pounds.

You may have help from a partner, family member or close friend in the early weeks, but eventually you will have to learn to feed both babies simultaneously, and it is much better to practise doing this when you do have someone else around.

If you are on your own doing the feed, it is also advisable to have nappies, wipes and a change of clothes for them close by too. If one or both of them decide to have a nappy explosion halfway through the feed, you won't want to go searching.

C-section babies

Babies born by Caesarean section can sometimes take a few days to 'get going' on the breast or bottle. When a baby is born naturally and the mother gives birth vaginally, the baby tends to have all or most of the amniotic fluid that she has swallowed in the uterus pushed out of her lungs as she passes through the birth canal.

With a baby born by C-section this doesn't happen as they get pulled out of the uterus rather unexpectedly to them, particularly if you have an elective section, where you aren't already in labour.

The recent amniotic fluid that they may have swallowed while happily floating around in the womb will therefore still be in their system.

Once born, the effect that it then has on the baby is to make them choke and gag frequently in the first few days after birth in an attempt to expel the excess fluid by vomiting it up. It is usually a greeny-yellow colour, like mucus, and can take up to a week to be fully out of their system.

You may find, particularly in the first couple of days after your C-section, that your baby just doesn't seem hungry or want to feed on the breast or bottle very regularly, but still seems settled and sleepy despite not eating a great deal.

This is because the fluid in her tummy is actually making her feel very full. Her hunger will depend on how much of a gulp of the amniotic fluid she had before being born. Some C-section babies have an appetite from day one, and feed fine, but it is also perfectly normal for others to take two to three days to begin to feed regularly, once she has cleared some of the fluid out of her tummy.

It's important that you still offer her a feed every three to four hours during the day though. If, despite a nappy change and lots of persevering, she still refuses to feed, then allow her to sleep for another hour and then repeat the waking up and trying to feed process again. Keep doing this every hour until she finally has a decent feed, after which you can allow her another three-to-four-hour stretch between feeds again.

I have had three C-sections. The first was an emergency one after a long labour, and my second and third were electives. My first baby took a good two days of persevering on the breast before he got hungry enough to feed regularly. I was almost ready to give up trying because I thought it was the breast he didn't like, but during those first two days he brought up a lot of mucus. I had a very good group of midwives who explained that it was very normal for C-section babies to behave this way. It's not very nice to watch as you feel so helpless. One minute they can be lying in the cot next to your bed sleeping, and the next you suddenly hear them gagging and choking.

The best thing to do is pick her up as quickly as possible, and sit her in the winding position on your lap. Pat her back and rub in the suggested winding rhythm described on page 105. It's wise to hold a muslin under her chin to catch anything she manages to vomit up. Sometimes a baby will gag and choke but swallow it back down again, which is another reason why it can sometimes take a few days to clear all of the mucus out of their system. I was very lucky with my second and third babies. Although they were very full of mucus, it didn't put them off feeding and they both breastfed well from the start.

It is wise to lie your baby on her side during this time in particular. You can place rolled-up towels or blankets behind and in front of her to hold her in position, and prevent her from rolling on to her front, where she may be at risk of suffocating. In my opinion all babies sleep better on their side in this position anyway – this is discussed in more detail in Chapter 5.

A baby who begins to vomit while lying on her back is at risk of choking on it as they are trying to expel it out of their mouth. The idea that a newborn baby will turn their head to the side as they begin to vomit to let it trickle out is ridiculous! Yet this was the information given to me when I questioned how safe it was to lay a C-section baby full of mucus on their back.

My middle child proved my point when I woke to find he had turned purple at 2 a.m. in the middle of a gagging/choking episode 24 hours after he was born. Luckily I woke to discover this and quickly sat him up and patted his back until he had recovered and calmed down. It really hit home to me how right I was to trust my instincts.

A baby panics if they begin to bring up a small amount of sick while sleeping. They will not just turn their head to the side for it to trickle out as is commonly suggested. Even an older baby will have the same reaction. I've laid older babies around six months of age down on a changing mat and they have still looked at me wide-eyed when they begin to vomit and start choking on it and swallowing it back down, until I pick them and help them spit it out by winding them.

As a baby gets older and has so much wind that they begin to be sick, they tend to cry at the same time, which prompts you to respond to them (particularly if they are now in a different room to you) and pick them up.

How to wind your baby

There are lots of ways to wind your baby in various positions, but the two main positions that most people use are pictured and described below.

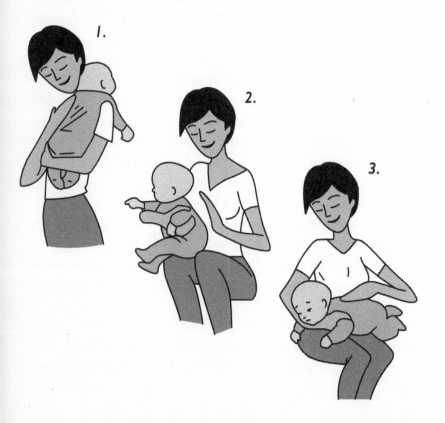

The first is by putting her up against your shoulder with her chest facing your chest (picture 1). Have one hand holding underneath her bottom to support her and use the other hand to pat and rub. The winding hand can also be used to support her head every now and then if she starts moving it around a lot and head-butting you.

As a guide, aim for 10 pats and 10 rubs. The pats should be aimed midway between the top of her shoulder blades and the middle of her back. Your pat needs to be quite firm to help the wind come up. Babies are very robust, even if they don't look it, and you won't hurt her with a firm pat! Generally the burp tends to come out as you are rubbing, so it is very important to follow the rhythm of 10 pats and 10 rubs to help the wind come up. If you do too much of one or the other it will make a difference to the time you have to spend winding your baby.

Another way of winding a baby is to sit her on your lap facing outwards (picture 2). Place your hand quite firmly under her chin and try to have her back as straight as possible. If her body is all scrunched up and huddled over, you will find it very difficult to get the wind out, and she may even vomit as the milk she has just drank is being squashed in her tummy – in this instance the only way is up! Use your other hand to do the 10 pats, 10 rubs rhythm.

Winding a baby lying on her tummy (picture 3) can sometimes work too, but it is more likely to make your baby vomit if she is prone to doing that regularly anyway.

I generally try the shoulder position first as I find it is a more comfortable position to wind a baby. If after five minutes like that I still haven't heard a burp then I switch to the sitting position winding method. If you still haven't heard a burp, and your baby continues to squirm, wriggle and look generally uncomfortable, then lie her down on the floor for a maximum of 60 seconds. If she really begins squirming and looking uncomfortable before the 60 seconds is up, then pick her up, put her over your shoulder and give her a little pat. This motion of lying a baby flat on their back is usually enough to make a burp come out when you pick them up again. You do have to get the timing right though because, if you leave her lying flat for too long and don't pick her up quick enough, then she will vomit! This is another learning curve where you will need to be guided by your baby. There will of course be a few times in the beginning where you don't get the timing right and she covers you and her in vomit!

Some babies will burp very easily after every feed and never suffer with any type of wind-related pain. Others will make you work really hard to get a burp out of them, and, even when they produce a couple of loud ones, they may still seem very uncomfortable. Almost all babies are fairly easy to wind for the first one to two weeks. It is at this point, around the age of two weeks, that you will begin to notice if your baby is going to be one who struggles with digestive and wind-related problems.

To be honest it is a complete luck of the draw if you get a baby who winds easily, or one who is going to struggle to bring it up and be rather uncomfortable because of it for the next few months. This is also true with whether you get a baby who is a little bit sicky, a lot sicky or never vomits a drop up, even among siblings.

CASE STUDY: My babies and wind

I thought my first baby was a bit of a sicky baby. He never really suffered from bad wind, but was generally a bit sick after most feeds. He fed well though and never had a problem with his weight gain so I didn't worry about it.

Once my second baby was born I realised that the sick that my first baby produced occasionally was nothing more than possetting compared to number two. He was a little vomit machine! He would sick up what looked like rivers of milk after **every** feed. Sometimes he wouldn't even have the manners to finish on the breast first and would just begin vomiting, and then quite happily latch back on as soon as he had been sick! He would get quite cross with me as I sat him up to clean me and him up, because all he wanted to do was carry on feeding! I had to always have a pile of bibs and muslins next to me as I breastfed him because it was guaranteed that we would use several at each feed. I couldn't lie him down flat for at least half an hour after a feed either, or he would vomit even more. Yet he always fed well, never had a problem burping and continued to put on almost a pound a week for the first eight to ten weeks, so I didn't worry. He gradually grew out of it as his digestive system got stronger and more developed, and by the age of six months he could finally wear an outfit without me worrying about him vomiting all over it!

My third child was different again. She was a bit hit-and-miss in terms of whether she would vomit or not. Some feeds she wouldn't spill a drop, whereas others we would have a large vomit that covered her and me. She always burped and winded very well during the day and didn't seem uncomfortable at all but from the age of around three to four weeks she began to be very unsettled at night with wind pain. Despite trying to wind her, a lot of the time we would be unable to get anything out, and the only thing that would calm her would be to lie on my or my husband's chest. This was only happening after the night feed, and between the hours of 5 and 7 a.m. she would wriggle and cry constantly unless she was sleeping upright on one of us. We decided to introduce Infacol for every feed as, although she seemed fine during the day, her wind was obviously building up to an uncomfortable level at night-time. Within a few days there was a vast improvement; she became much more settled at night and was happier to go back into her basket after the night feed again. She continued to posset and be sick at some feeds but, like my other two, always put on between half a pound and a pound per week, so I didn't worry about it. When we weaned her off her night feed at nine weeks she became much more settled at night, as her body didn't have to deal with the extra milk intake.

There are things you can do to help ease the pain of wind like changing feeding positions. There are also over-the-counter products, like Infacol that you can buy to help control and keep on top of the wind build up. There are also similar products called Dentinox and gripe water too, although gripe can only be given from one month, whereas the other two products can be given from birth. Unfortunately there is nothing that will give you a magic cure though. It is just something that you and your baby will have to try to work around until she gets older and her digestive system becomes stronger. As she grows her whole body stretches out more too so that she is not in that scrunched up foetal position all the time. This also makes it easier for her to burp and release wind.

Trumping or farting is also a form of releasing wind, so if your baby isn't really a big burper, but has a lot of bottom wind and seems quite happy after a feed, then she is probably releasing it this way!

Having a very windy baby is totally different to having a baby with reflux or colic. Some people are too quick to jump to the conclusion that their baby has one of these, as opposed to just being a very windy baby. It will still be very painful at times and terribly uncomfortable for your baby if she suffers from bad wind, but be careful not to confuse the things.

Colic, reflux and hiccups

There are differences between all of these things but they tend to all get confused with each other. The structure of your baby's feeds and the foods and liquid you drink if breastfeeding can make a lot of difference to how windy your baby is, or how 'colicky' she behaves. Babies who are fed too often and get used to snack feeding will be much more unsettled and more likely to suffer from excess wind or colic.

Below I have given a description of each and information on how you can help relieve symptoms.

Colic

Colic is a term used to describe uncontrollable crying in a healthy baby. NHS Choice's definition of the condition is as follows:

Colic is the medical term for excessive, frequent crying in a baby who appears to be otherwise healthy and well fed. It is a poorly understood yet common condition and affects around one in five babies. A baby with colic may have several crying outbursts a day, a few times a week. The crying pattern usually begins within the first few weeks of life but often stops by the time the baby is four months old, and by six months at the latest.

Research suggests that chocolate, coffee, tea, cola and onions are among the foods that a breastfeeding mother should avoid as they act as stimulants. You could also try a period of eliminating dairy, nuts, soy or citrus fruits one at a time over a period of one week, to evaluate if there is any improvement to the baby's behaviour.

In my experience the majority of babies that display symptoms of colic, are being snack fed.

Snack feeding plays a huge part in giving your baby excess wind, which can become so bad they will then display colic symptoms where they cry continuously, draw their legs up in pain and seem genuinely unhappy. When a baby is snack fed every couple of hours, then their feed will have less time to digest in their tummy, and some wind and air bubbles may still remain from the previous feed. Giving them more milk on top of the air bubble that is already sitting in their tummy not only means that they are more likely to vomit but also that you are trapping the air bubble. This is then much harder to get out and your baby will cry, as it can cause them pain. Repeated snack feeding adds to this, ending up in a vicious circle.

It is my belief that structuring your baby's feeds from the start prevents this from happening, and none of the babies I have worked with has ever gone through stages of continuous inconsolable crying. I would be very worried if they did, but on the whole I believe it is something that can be prevented.

If your baby takes a full feed and has a structured feeding pattern where she sticks to the times stated and doesn't snack feed but still seems unhappy, then the problem may be due to very bad wind that has got trapped and is causing colic pain. I would first of all try an infant colic remedy at each feed – Infacol, Dentinox or gripe water – to see if that relieves symptoms. The active ingredient (Simeticone) contained in these products helps the little trapped gas bubbles join in to bigger bubbles, which your baby can more easily bring up as wind.

Milk, infant formula, breast milk and other dairy products contain a type of sugar called lactose. Those who suffer from lactose intolerance are unable to properly digest this type of sugar in their bodies and this will also cause them pain. Research at Guy's Hospital in 1999 linked one of the causes of colic to lactose intolerance. Babies born with a lactose intolerance may also vomit after a feed and not be gaining a vast amount of weight.

A key difference between the symptoms of colic and lactose intolerance is that the lactose-intolerant baby suffers from diarrhoea. The osmotic pressure generated by lactose and lactic acid in the stomach produces an influx of water, leading to a swollen abdomen and acidic diarrhoea. If you do suspect that your baby is lactose intolerant then consult your family doctor for advice and confirmatory testing, rather than attempting to self-diagnose. They will be qualified to advise you on what action to take next.

A formula-fed baby will need to be changed to milk that doesn't contain lactose to solve the problem. This will come on prescription from your doctor as it cannot be bought from the supermarket. A mother who is breastfeeding her baby would need to cut lactose out of her diet completely. This is much easier said than done – as one of the mothers I worked for found out!

CASE STUDY: David's experience

David was solely breastfed, with expressed milk given in a bottle for the 10:30 p.m. feed. He was doing very well and by six weeks was feeding on schedule and sleeping well at night between feeds. He would take the bottle very well at 10:30 p.m. and drink between 4 and 6fl oz (120 and 180ml). He was still being breastfed at night because his mother, Sarah, wasn't able to produce enough expressed milk on top of his daily feeding needs to be able to give two expressed feeds. She didn't want to resort to formula either for the 10:30 p.m. feed, as both of David's older sisters had suffered from dairy and lactose intolerance. At just over six weeks he began getting very upset during feed times – crying, drawing his legs up and being very difficult to breastfeed. He was Sarah's third baby, and her two older girls had both suffered from various feeding, issues: tongue tie, dairy intolerance, reflux, weight loss due to poor feeding, etc., so his mum had been waiting for David to follow suit and develop issues too. Her paediatrician had warned her that intolerances were usually genetic. It was such a shame he began to develop feeding issues as he had been doing so well, and we were beginning to hope he hadn't been affected.

He began to struggle to take in his regular amount of milk at each feed, as he was in so much pain. He was always perfectly happy to wait until the next planned feed time before he had any more milk, despite only taking a reduced feed. The day feeds continued in the same way, and the only feed that David seemed to take well without any fussing was the 3–4 a.m. night feed. He would be so relaxed at this time that he would happily take both breasts, as he had built up a real hunger due to the scrappy feeds he had been having all day. He would also settle much better afterwards and sleep well with a happy tummy.

We continued to let him have this feed, as it was the only one where he would take a good amount, and after discussion we agreed that Sarah should cut out any dairy products, such as cow's milk, she was consuming, to see if that helped. Within a week David was coping well – taking some feeds better than others, but feeding had improved. However, we found that there were times where we would have two to three days where he would regress badly. Looking back to what his mum had eaten the 24–48 hours previously it seemed even the slightest amount of dairy would give him very bad pain and cause him to struggle to feed for days. Things like eating a piece of cake made with a small amount of milk or having a small square of chocolate would have a profound effect on him for two to three days! He would fuss and scream during feeds and wouldn't poo for days, which made him even more uncomfortable.

After taking David to a paediatrician his mother was advised to cut out any form of dairy completely if she wanted to continue breastfeeding. She was told that the lack of soiled nappies and the fact that his 6 p.m. feed was generally his worst one of the day was very normal for a baby suffering from reflux caused by a dairy intolerance because it affects the whole digestive system. It is always worse when the tummy is full at the end of the day and a tiny amount of dairy can throw a baby off their regular feeds for 48 hours or so.

David was put on two different types of medication to try to help relieve the symptoms of reflux and colic. This was combined with a strict diet for his mother. Acidic foods worsen reflux too so a nursing mother has to eat as though she herself has reflux. There may be certain feeds that a baby will happily tolerate but it is purely trial and error. Particular foods to avoid are wine, tomatoes, chocolate, citrus, cow's milk, vinegars, fried foods and fatty meats.

He was also given a prescription for infant formula milk that didn't contain any cow's milk.

David's feeding did begin to improve once he began the medication, but Sarah was still breastfeeding and he continued to have bad spells lasting a couple of days occasionally, due to foods in her diet that caused a reaction. As it was very difficult for his mother to pinpoint what foods in her diet were causing him the pain, she decided to begin to wean him on to formula. This was a challenge in itself, as all the feeding issues meant David often refused point blank to take the bottle at all.

By now he was four and a half months old. I had moved on to my next booked contract but Sarah and I were in contact most days via email discussing David's progress. He still continued to have his night feed, as Sarah was loath to take that one away too soon, as she was well aware that at times it was his most relaxed feed that he enjoyed the most. He was gradually changed over to the prescription formula for his day feeds and then weaned at just over five months by recommendation of his paediatrician. After a few weeks he was eating a variety of home-made fruit and vegetables, and drinking the new formula from a bottle. He was, however, still waking at night out of habit and Sarah continued to breastfeed him when he did, as it was the quickest way to settle him back down. He had various coughs, colds and ear infections over the winter months too, which set them back by a week or so each time, and understandably made it harder for Sarah to be too strict with him while he was unwell.

Finally, at just over six months, David was over all of his bugs, the medication was working well and Sarah decided it was time to tackle the night feeding. He was taking a good amount of solids and formula during the day so, after discussion, we came to the conclusion that using the cry-it-out method was our only option.

This involves going in and checking your baby for wind initially when she first wakes up crying. If you pick her up and she doesn't have any wind then you lie her back down and then leave her to 'cry it out'. You can go back in and check on her by looking at her over the resulting period of time after the initial pick up, but you shouldn't let her see you again and you have to refrain from picking her up again after the first time. It is a method that not all mothers are happy to try, as understandably listening to your baby cry, and not responding to it, is an extremely hard thing for any mother to do. You have to be a pretty strong person to be able to do it, or have tried every other method available and be left with no other option. Depending on the age of the baby, the crying can potentially go on for a very long period of time – up to an hour in some cases.

As Sarah had tried various other methods, she felt that the cry-it-out method was now the only thing that would work on David to stop him waking and expecting to be nursed back to sleep during the night. I had to agree. He was over six months old now and definitely didn't need a night feed; he was waking purely due to habit. If Sarah went in to him and picked him up he would nuzzle her and cry until she gave in, so she knew herself that she had to break that habit of even giving him the temptation.

The first night he woke at 2:30 a.m. After going in and checking for wind Sarah laid him back down and walked out. He cried on and off for over an hour before finally giving in and going back to sleep. He then woke again around 5 a.m. I had advised Sarah that she should go in and check on him during the second waking (to make sure he wasn't stuck in an awkward position etc.), but not to allow him to see her or to pick him up. She did this – he was fine – so she walked back out and he cried for 40 minutes and then slept until 7 a.m. when she went in to wake him. He woke very happy and smiley, which reassured Sarah that she wasn't the bad mother she felt like for leaving him to cry and that he still responded to seeing her in a good way!

I had also advised Sarah that she should be the one to go in and wake him, rather than allowing him to wake up again crying and then get him up. This would send him the wrong message. The cry-it-out method is all about teaching a baby that you are in control of their sleep and not them. It is always important to get to them as they are first waking up and still rolling around and gurgling or chatting. If they are still asleep when you go in first thing in the morning or at any other sleep time, then you can rouse them by opening the curtains and talking to them to wake them up. You are usually then greeted with a lovely smile, which is the perfect way for them to wake up.

If you only ever wait until your baby cries before going in to get her in the morning then she will learn to associate crying with her way to get you to come, and will always wake up crying. This isn't a very nice way for her to wake and it's not really something you will enjoy hearing every morning either. In a way it kind of starts both of your days off really badly.

The cry-it-out method is explained fully in Chapter 5.

The second night David again woke a couple of times but cried for a much shorter time. Things continued to improve over the following few nights until he happily began sleeping through until 6 a.m. most mornings and would then play in his cot until Sarah went in at 7 a.m.

It was a very long haul to get David's sleeping established, mainly because of the intolerances and resulting colic and reflux, which meant he developed bad associations with sleep. He got there in the end though, and finally sleeps very well, much to his mother's enormous pleasure after the long period of sleep-deprived nights!

Reflux

Over the past 15 years many thousands of fussy babies have been given medicine in the belief that their colic was caused by painful acid reflux, so called gastro-oesophageal reflux disease (GORD).

There are very important differences between gastro-oesophageal reflux (GOR) and GORD when describing reflux in babies.

Reflux is caused by a baby having a 'floppy' or under-developed sphincter valve at the top of their diaphragm. This valve is supposed to be one way and only allow food to pass down the oesophagus (food pipe) and into the stomach, and not allow it to come back up again. In some babies the valve action isn't as strong because the sphincter action of the diaphragm isn't fully developed. It gradually gets stronger over the first year of a baby's life and her chance of developing reflux decreases.

GOR refers to the passage of stomach contents coming into the oesophagus. It sometimes enters the throat and is brought up as a small or large vomit. More than 50 per cent of babies will experience some reflux once or more a day and will be perfectly happy from feed to feed despite their vomiting. This is a normal occurrence and one they will outgrow with time. Feeding in the correct position and introducing solid food will also help ease the amount of vomit they produce, as will not laying her down flat immediately after a feed.

Symptoms of GORD

Over the past five years various studies have proved that GORD rarely causes infant crying. Even crying during feeding and crying accompanied by writhing and back arching is rarely related to acid reflux unless the baby also has:

- *Poor weight gain*
- *Large amounts of vomiting (more than five times per day, although reflux babies do not always vomit)*
- *A habit of fussing or refusing feeds – but will suck on a dummy. Reflux babies very quickly learn to associate feeding with pain*
- *Occasional blood in her stools*
- *Very unsettled sleep at night. This one is more difficult to pinpoint as all small babies wake in the night*

In contrast, GORD is not normal and will cause your baby a lot of pain and discomfort. This is caused by your baby's stomach acid mixing with the milk she has just swallowed, then travelling back up her oesophagus. If as an adult you have ever experienced heartburn then this is the closest way to describe the pain it causes in a baby. Unfortunately babies cannot tell you what they are feeling, so you will have to look out for various other symptoms.

Babies with reflux will not be happy or comfortable lying on their back on a flat surface. The positions that work for them are to be upright, lying on an adult's chest with their chest facing yours; or propped upright on a cushion or V-pillow on their front. Sometimes they are also happy to lie on their side, but, again, propped up and not completely flat. Until you treat the reflux and can control the symptoms effectively they will never be happy to lie flat on their back to sleep, as it will cause them too much pain.

Both GOR and GORD are more common in premature babies as their systems are less mature. See your doctor if you think that your baby is suffering from either of these conditions. It can help if you can take a diary of feeds and periods of crying to give your doctor a clear idea of what is happening, so that they can advise on various treatments.

If you are breastfeeding it may be worth cutting cow's milk from your diet completely to see if this has a positive effect on your baby. In up to 40 per cent of cases, cow's milk allergy or intolerance is found to be the underlying cause of reflux. You could try this before you see your GP.

If your baby is formula fed then you can ask your doctor about trying a hypo-allergenic formula for a couple of weeks to see if that helps. These infant formulas are specifically designed for infants and toddlers with severe cow's milk protein allergies and/ or multiple food protein allergies.

Your doctor may also suggest you try an antacid such as Gaviscon. Your doctor will prescribe this with directions on the dose and how to give for bottle- and breastfed babies. If the antacid doesn't help, then your baby may need to be prescribed some reflux medication to relieve symptoms. In my experience the babies that have gone on to this medication have shown a vast improvement even within the first 48 hours, and are like a completely different baby after a week or more on the medication. You may still have good days and bad days in terms of how windy or sicky your baby is, but this is normal anyway even for a baby that doesn't suffer from reflux, and doesn't mean that the medication is not working. The older your baby gets, and the more developed her valve becomes, the better her symptoms will get. Babies generally do not need to be weaned off the medication. As she gets older and begins to put on more weight the dose she was initially given for her weight begins to become so minimal for her increased weight that it will cease to have an effect anyway. Any improvements she makes as she grows will be due to her body becoming more developed and her digestive system dealing with any milk she drinks in a more effective way.

CASE STUDY: Alix and Isla's experience

Alix and Isla were the first-ever set of twins that I worked with. They were born at 35 weeks gestation and after a week or so in the special care baby unit were well enough to come home. They had been established on a three-hourly feeding pattern in the hospital, which we continued. They were given either expressed breast milk or formula in their bottles to drink, depending on how much EBM we had available.

Isla was a very easy baby. She always fed well and settled between feeds. Alix, on the other hand, struggled from the start. He would always be very windy and uncomfortable at feed times, and wasn't great at going down after a feed. He was hardly ever sick but preferred to be kept upright or propped on something after a feed. We put him on Infacol to see if that would help initially but I warned the mum that if we didn't see any improvement then she should take him to their GP as I was worried he had reflux. The Infacol didn't help – he still continued to cry a lot during and after feeds and the nights were spent with him propped up on one of our chests, as it was the only position that gave him any respite at all. Even that didn't always work!

His mother, Pip, took him to their GP, who gave him a prescription for Gaviscon to try first. After a week on this and still no improvement Pip took him back to the GP, who finally gave in and prescribed some medicine for reflux called Ranitidine. Within a week he was like a different baby – much happier during feed times and not suffering with huge amounts of pain afterwards. By this time he was about six weeks old and had understandably developed some bad sleep associations of being held a lot to get to sleep, and needing to be frequently resettled. This was unavoidable: we had to do whatever worked until his reflux was being controlled.

We all worked hard over the following couple of weeks to structure his sleeping pattern a bit better and encourage him to go down for a sleep without being held, and his days and nights improved dramatically.

His twin Isla had been a model baby throughout all this time while we were getting Alix sorted out, but at the age of eight weeks, she began vomiting huge amounts at every feed, and crying in pain afterwards. After four days of this Pip called her doctor and he advised her to begin giving the reflux medication to Isla too.

Her vomiting then settled down after a few days of being on the medication and we were able to drop their night feed and get them sleeping through the night by the age of 12 weeks.

As these twins proved, reflux can be present from a very early age, but it is also possible for it to develop a bit later on when your baby is already a couple of months old.

Hiccups

Hiccups are very common in small babies and are perfectly normal; they aren't usually cause for concern. They are most likely to occur just after a feed, or when she gets excited (giggling or laughing a lot can cause them when she's old enough to do that). Hiccups have nothing to do with breathing. They are caused by sudden contractions of the diaphragm, caused by irritation or stimulation of that muscle. If your baby used to get them regularly in the womb, particularly at the end of your pregnancy, then you may find that she suffers from them regularly after every feed, every day for the first month or so. All three of my children did, but it improved after the first four weeks or so. Some babies are just more prone to them. Hiccups are considered harmless unless they are persistent enough to interfere with regular feeding and sleeping.

Sucking is usually the best way to get rid of them, either on a dummy or the breast or bottle. If you are in the middle of a feed and your baby gets the hiccups after a winding session then try to encourage her to continue feeding. Continued sucking through the hiccups will mean that they will gradually fade away. If your baby refuses to feed while still hiccupping then you could encourage her to suck on a dummy to get rid of them. If you were to just wait for them to go during a feed, then you could be waiting a long time and your baby will lose interest in finishing her feed.

Babies with gastro-oesophageal reflux disease (GORD) may tend to hiccup more frequently, accompanied by spitting up, vomiting and irritability. This should be mentioned to your GP, as should very frequent bouts of uncontrollable hiccups – particularly if your baby is over one year.

Growth spurts

These occur roughly around seven to ten days, two to three weeks, six weeks, twelve weeks and sixteen weeks, give or take a few days either side of these ages. They generally last two to three days. During this period of time your baby will probably want a top-up between some of her feeds, despite taking a full breast or bottle feed earlier and possibly even spending longer on the breast at each feed or want extra milk from the bottle.

If you find that she is showing signs of being hungry, won't settle with the dummy to pacify her, and you still have an hour or more before the next planned full feed time, then it is okay to feed her.

I would advise though that you treat the feed purely as a 'top-up' and attempt to get away with a short snack feed of up to 10 minutes on the breast or a 2fl oz (60ml) bottle feed. Then do your full feed at the usual time that you were planning to anyway.

This ensures that you are always aiming to get your baby back on track again.

I would never tell any of the mothers I work for not to offer their baby a top-up if they genuinely believe that she is hungry and needs an extra feed. A baby who is genuinely hungry will not be pacified by a dummy or being walked around and distracted. When they are that hungry, particularly during growth spurts, it is important that you allow them the benefit of the doubt. I would recommend that you top-up as much as your baby requires during and in between the daytime feeds, which should hopefully ensure they stick to needing only one feed around 3–4 a.m. during the core night hours.

In loose terms you are still demand feeding your baby from the day they are born because you will never refuse them a feed if they are genuinely hungry. However you are also trying to work towards a routine from the day they are born, and encourage her to feed at particular times, which remain the same every day.

Changes to feeding as your baby gets older

As your baby gets older she will become more efficient at feeding and therefore empty the breast or bottle more quickly. She will still be getting the same amount, or probably even more as her appetite increases and your breasts also increase the supply they are producing, but she won't need to spend as long on the breast to get it.

This is very normal, so don't worry if she drops to 15–20 minutes on the first breast, even if she had been previously having 30 minutes or more. Do your checks to ensure she has reached the hind milk and make sure your breast feels pretty empty. If it does then you can swap her on to the second breast. As long as she continues to go the distance between feeds and put on a regular amount of weight then she must be getting enough milk to satisfy her daily needs. Regardless of the reduced time she spends on the first breast as she gets more efficient at feeding, her total time should always be made up of a longer period on the first breast than the second. If you find that she begins spending equal amounts on both breasts, then it's a good idea to encourage her to spend a longer period of time on the first breast instead, as it's highly likely that she isn't getting enough hind milk from the first breast. It is very normal for one breast to be bigger than the other and be producing a more plentiful supply. You will also notice that your baby prefers the breast with the bigger supply. It's very important that you still continue to feed evenly from each breast though by alternating the breast that you begin each feed from and pumping off any milk not used by your baby, and saving it to use at a later date. You will probably find that your baby is able to empty the breast with the lower supply in a much quicker time and may even want to spend longer on the second breast on the occasions where you start the feed on the breast with the lower supply. Again this is perfectly normal and fine to let her do. Most babies have a preference for one breast or the other; it just means you have to work a bit harder to encourage her to still feed from the other one to encourage a good milk supply.

CASE STUDY: Stress, breastfeeding and me

The impact that being stressed or upset can have on your milk supply was really hit home to me one evening. My husband and I had been having a disagreement over something minor. It was the end of the evening and I was very tired after a busy day with a small baby and a toddler to look after. I knew I was also going to be up again that night and was having a very hormonal day anyway, and my hubby winding me up wasn't helping. It got to 10:15 p.m. and we still hadn't resolved our differences but I knew I needed to go and express before my baby boy woke for his feed. Usually I would pump while sitting in front of the TV, relaxing and chatting to my husband, but I was so annoyed with him I just got the pump and decided to go upstairs to our bedroom to do it. Every other night for the past couple of weeks I had been able to express off a total of between 8 and 10fl oz (240–300ml) between both breasts. I began pumping as usual, but my let down didn't come as quickly as it normally did in the first 20–30 seconds. I continued pumping off the first breast but after two to three minutes I still hadn't had a let down and my nipple was beginning to get sore. I decided to swap to the other breast and then come back to that one rather than keep pumping and getting nowhere, as I could feel myself getting stressed and knew that wouldn't be helping matters. However, the same happened on the other breast too, and I just couldn't relax enough to get a let down. I knew in my head why it was all happening and that because I was stressed due to the argument with my husband, and tired and tearful that the milk refused to come. However, that didn't make it any easier to deal with! I decided to have a break and then try pumping again in half an hour. The same still happened though and I couldn't produce more than half an ounce in total from both breasts.

The next day was a much better. Hubby and I had made up and were on good terms again, so I was very relaxed when it came to expressing that night. I had my usual spot on the sofa in front of the TV and began pumping. I must admit I was a little worried about what would happen, and whether I would produce any milk this time, but everything was fine and I pumped my usual 8–10fl oz (240–300ml) that I had been doing the previous couple of weeks. Relief washed over me and I was very happy everything was back to normal. It really made me realise though how much an impact tiredness and stress can have on your ability to produce a good amount of milk.

Introducing a regular bottle to a breastfed baby.

Breastfeeding mothers are often actively discouraged from offering their baby a bottle at all. They are told by a large number of healthcare professionals, which include health visitors and midwives, that giving a baby a bottle (whether it is expressed breast milk – EBM – or formula) will confuse their baby and put her off the idea of breastfeeding. This can scare mothers, particularly first-time ones, who really want to be able to breastfeed successfully. The unfortunate thing is they then refrain from offering a bottle for so long that when they eventually do, at the age of four, five or six months, or in some cases even later, their baby understandably refuses to take one at all.

My recommendation is that a breastfed baby is offered a bottle of EBM on a daily basis from the age of two to three weeks. Once breastfeeding is established, which usually takes between 7 and 14 days, and the mother has a good milk supply, a breastfed baby will *never* prefer a bottle rather than the breast, and will certainly *never* go off the breast completely. I am not just assuming this, which is what a lot of people do when telling new mothers that their baby will probably go off the breast if they give them a bottle, I know this to be true for a fact!

I have worked with hundreds of babies, and every single one of them that has been breastfed solely from day one, including own three children, has been given at least one (but usually two) bottles of either EBM or formula from the age of 7–14 days old – and *not one* of them has gone off breastfeeding at all! In fact, many babies will happily take the breast immediately after a full bottle-feed as a form of comfort, just because they enjoy the closeness with their mummy.

You will instinctively know when your baby is 'established on the breast.' She will be latching on well each time without too

---

Tip

For your baby to accept the bottle happily without any fuss or problems with the transition it needs to be done by the age of four weeks at the latest. For every week you leave it after this age your baby is less likely to be interested in the idea of taking milk from anything other than the breast. If you are happy with this scenario and would like to continue solely breastfeeding your baby without ever getting her established on to a bottle, that is fine. This section has been written for mothers who may want or need to get their babies established on to a bottle to make things more practical and less of a strain when they need to go back to work. It's also helpful to know that a baby will happily take a bottle of milk if you want to leave your baby with a family member or close friend for a period of time that involves feeding.

much fuss and taking regular feeds. Once you get to this point, which usually happens by the time they are around 14 days old, then you can introduce a bottle.

I have had calls from countless mothers whose babies have been completely breastfed from day one and never been offered a bottle. The mother then reaches the stage where they are almost completely tied to their baby, because the only form of milk she will accept is directly from the breast. This means she can never go out and leave her baby with a family member or close friend for more than a couple of hours at a time, as she needs to be available for feeding.

From a practical point of view it is good to get your baby used to a bottle from an early age if you are planning on going back to work after a period of maternity leave at home. For the majority of families today, it is necessary for both the mother and father to work, even if only part-time hours for one parent.

A lot of parents are lulled into a false sense of security over how easy it is to get a baby to take a bottle later on, when it becomes a necessity that they need to take one, due to work commitments etc. Unfortunately it is never that easy and she may fight you tooth and nail and refuse to feed from it every step of the way.

The worst part is that once you reach this stage the only way to get a baby to begin taking milk from a bottle is to go 'cold turkey' on the breast. A baby will never starve themselves and will always give in and eat once they get hungry enough. You will need to offer a bottle of expressed milk every couple of hours during the day – without relenting, and offering the breast, if she refuses to drink from the bottle. Eventually she will not be able to refuse to drink from the bottle any longer, as her natural instinct to eat will take over. The fact that you are offering breast milk initially will help a great deal as the taste will still be familiar to her. If you don't have enough breast milk to offer her in the bottle then it is fine to use formula instead. For the first 24 hours you are likely to have a lot of wasted milk. You will need to throw away any milk she has refused after trying to get her to feed for a maximum of an hour. The next time that you offer a bottle it will need to be a fresh feed with new breast milk or formula.

If you are trying to get your baby to take a bottle for practical reasons – work-related, or to give yourself a bit more freedom in going out without her – then you will need to pump milk from your breasts at what would be your baby's usual feed times. This will ensure that your body still produces milk if you would like to continue with breastfeeding, but are just trying to introduce a regular bottle.

It is very important that you don't offer your baby the breast again too quickly, or she will refuse the bottle again if she knows there is a better offer on the table! Wait until she has drunk at least three bottle-feeds before offering the breast at the next feed. The feed after that should then be a bottle, and if she takes that happily without any fuss, then you can begin to alternate breast and bottle. I would advise that you continue with a minimum of two feeds per day as bottle-feeds, so that you minimise the risk of her going off the bottle again.

If you are moving her to the bottle because your breast milk supply has dwindled despite efforts to revive it, then, if she has never been offered a bottle before, I would still suggest you follow the above method. You may find that you can still manage to do a couple of breastfeeds per day if you supplement the others with formula. See advice on page 135 for details on how to wean your baby from breast to bottle when you would like to stop breastfeeding all together.

Some mothers prefer to go straight from solely breastfeeding to offering cow's milk in a sippy cup or beaker once their baby is over a year old, without the need to use bottles at all. This is absolutely fine too if it is practical for you not to be apart from your baby for any length of time. You can continue solely breastfeeding without introducing bottles for as long as you and your baby are enjoying it.

What is the best time of day to introduce a bottle-feed?

It is best to offer your baby a bottle at the 10:30 p.m. feed and the 3–4 a.m. night feed, depending on whether you would like your baby to have one or two bottles per 24 hours. Initially, as a first bottle-feed, I would advise you to offer your baby a bottle at the 10:30 p.m. feed. If you can manage to pump off some of your own breast milk to put in a bottle and offer your baby, this would be ideal, rather than formula. You may already have some stored in the freezer from the first few days of engorgement, if you managed to express any excess milk.

Defrosting EBM

To defrost a freezer bag of EBM you stand the bag in a bowl of boiling water with a sterilised bottle ready. As the iced milk melts, open the bag and transfer the liquid to the bottle immediately by pouring it into it from the bag. Repeat this every time a little bit of the iced milk melts until the freezer bag is empty. It is important that you transfer the milk as soon as it melts, so that the liquid doesn't begin to heat up, as baby milk cannot be reheated more than once. Place the cold, defrosted EBM in the bottle in the fridge until needed.

If you do not already have some EBM in the freezer but would prefer your baby to stay on breast milk rather than formula, here are some guidelines for how and when to express:

• Express 1–2fl oz (30–60ml) off the first breast (amount depends on how full you feel with milk) *before* you put your baby to the breast. This will not take milk away from your baby, and it will actually help her to get to the hind milk much faster. You may find that she doesn't need to spend a full 30 minutes or her usual time on the first breast, as she will empty it quicker because you have expressed. You can also express an ounce or so off the second breast before putting your baby on. By pumping first and putting her to the breast afterwards, she will encourage your breasts to produce more milk with her sucking at the end of the feed. Baby's sucking can always extract much more milk from the breast, even if you can't seem to get any more with the pump.

- Express during your first two to three feeds of the day – so the 7:30 a.m., 10:30 a.m. and (only if you still feel full) the 2:30 p.m. Place this expressed milk in a freezer bag or sterile container, and put in the body of the fridge.
- You can mix milk together produced over the same 24-hour period. However you do need to make sure that that they are the same temperature when you mix them – so not one that's cold in the fridge and one still warm and only just expressed. Store them in separate containers in the fridge until both are at the same temperature, and then you can mix them together.
- If for some reason you, are unable to express enough milk to give your baby EBM then formula is fine. Speak to your health visitor about the current recommended infant formula milk that is most similar to breast milk.

Top tip

This is a fantastic opportunity for your partner to get involved with feeding, and have some special bonding time with your little one. My husband was counting down the days until the first 'big bottle-feed' with all three of our babies, as do many dads. They become very proud that they are able to play a more active role with their new baby. I can tell you first-hand that, from a mother's point of view, it is just amazing to watch them together for the first time.

As a first bottle-feed I would suggest making up a feed of between 3 and 4fl oz (90 and 120ml). After the first few times that she has had a bottle, you will have more of an idea of the amount she is capable of drinking, and can increase the amount accordingly.

Doing the actual feed

Please see the bottle-feeding section (page 92) for how to sterilise and make up bottles of formula, and how to heat milk.

With a baby who has been breastfed entirely in the days/weeks before you offer a bottle, I would recommend that you heat her bottled milk to a nice warm temperature for her to drink. Breast milk comes out at body temperature, so this will be what she will be used to, and it is unlikely she will like the idea of drinking cold milk or even milk at room temperature. By offering her the milk in her bottle at a similar temperature, you will make the transition easier for her.

As her mother, she is more likely to fuss on the bottle when *you* are feeding her, because she knows you have something better to offer her directly from the breast. It is better to get your partner or another family member to do the bottle-feed the first few times, until she is used to it. It is also then important that you give the bottle to her every now and again, just so that you know she will take it from you.

You may find it easier to prop her up on some cushions to bottle-feed her, rather than holding her cradled in your arms. She will be used to this position with you for breastfeeding, so using a different position when you bottle-feed her will make the difference easier for her, as she won't have a breast so close to her head.

- Tease her mouth with the teat, as you would with your nipple when breastfeeding. Let her root around and then as she tastes the warm milk you will find she naturally begins to suck and draw the bottle teat into her mouth.
- Be guided by your baby in terms of when she needs to stop and be winded. See earlier information for more details on winding and positions to use (page 104).

> **Top tip**
>
> As she is drinking, move the teat to the side to break the sucking suction every 30 seconds or so but without actually removing the teat from her mouth. This will stop her sucking the teat completely flat and taking in too much excess air. It will also encourage her to keep drinking even when she is sleepy.

- While your partner is bottle-feeding your baby you will need to express the milk from your breasts at this time, or if you are doing the bottle-feed yourself then ideally express beforehand, or after the feed if you haven't had time. It is important that you empty both breasts fully at this time using the pump. The milk that you get can then be frozen or used for a night-feed bottle or the following evening's 10:30 p.m. feed.

- Once your baby has finished taking her milk you can also offer her the breast (once you have expressed though), if she is still looking for a bit of comfort and still seems unsettled. She will still be able to get some milk from your breast, even if you felt you got all there was using the breast pump. This extra milk that she takes from you will fill her up a bit more before what will hopefully be her longest stretch of sleep, and will also encourage your breasts to produce even more. She may not always want or need this breast top-up after the bottle, but if she is still awake after the bottle-feed then it's worth offering.

The other feed that many mothers – including myself – change to a bottle-feed of EBM, is the 3–4 a.m. night feed. This is for a number of reasons:

- It is quicker to bottle-feed the same amount of milk. She is also more likely to settle quicker with a bottle-feed because she will feel full in a shorter space of time. This means you end up getting back to bed faster, and any chance of extra sleep should not be dismissed in these early months!

- It is easier to bottle-feed a sleepy baby than it is to breastfeed her. You can just wiggle the bottle teat every now and then to stimulate her to continue sucking and take a full feed. This will make her less likely to wake again a couple of hours later, looking for more milk. You tend to need quite a bit of 'audience participation' when breastfeeding.

  If your baby wakes asking for a feed but then falls asleep at the breast after 10 minutes of feeding, and is far too sleepy to want to take any more, she is guaranteed to want more a couple of hours later, because she has only taken the fore milk. As discussed earlier, snack feeding is a very easy habit to fall into but not one that is good or healthy for either of you in the long term. It is also very easy for your baby to come to rely on the breast as a prop to get her back to sleep again. Every time she comes into a light sleep she will look to the breast for comfort once she is in the habit of snack feeding at night. This will be another habit that becomes more and more difficult to break the longer it continues.

- A lot of parents enjoy the reassurance of being able to see and control the amount of milk their baby has in the night. It also makes it a lot easier to wean the baby off their middle-of-the-night feed.

- There is no need to express in the middle of the night as your baby has the bottle of expressed milk – although you can if you want to try to keep your maximum milk supply, particularly in the first few weeks. It depends how quickly you are able to express.

CASE STUDY: The early weeks with my daughter

When my daughter was small I would have a bottle of expressed milk ready for her, which I had bought upstairs and placed in a cool bag in her room. When I heard her waking in the night I would quickly go and place her bottle of EBM in the bottle warmer and then pump off 2fl oz (60ml) milk from each breast using the sterilised pump that I had also placed in the cool bag. Luckily I was always able to express very easily and quickly, and would be done in five minutes flat, by which time her bottle would be ready, and I would go and fetch her from the Moses basket to bottle-feed her. If she had started crying while I was gone my husband would pick her up until I came back again and relieved him of his duties so that he could go back to sleep again! I only expressed for the first few weeks while my supply was building up, and then once she dropped her night feed around 10 weeks I didn't bother any more.

Top tip

It is perfectly fine to drop one feed per 24 hours without your milk supply being affected. Ideally you can make the one to drop the night feed, which can be changed to a bottle of EBM. As mentioned above, if you would like to express while your baby is having this feed as a bottle, that is perfectly fine. However you don't have to. What you can do to compensate for not breastfeeding or expressing in the night, is to express a little off both breasts first thing in the morning **before** your baby is put to the breast. This will encourage your breasts to still continue to produce the excess milk, and your baby will be happy to get on to the nice fatty hind milk much quicker without being drowned in lots of fore milk when your breasts are so full.

You will still need to express at the 10–11 p.m. feed if your baby is having a bottle though. Your breasts will still continue to produce a good supply of milk with one dropped feed, however if you dropped two feeds, e.g., the 10:30 p.m. and the night feed, and didn't express the milk off, you would notice your milk supply take a hit within a few days.

I know that many mothers' biggest fear is that if their baby has too many bottles in a row that she will be put off the breast the next time that it is offered. Please don't panic or worry about this. Once breastfeeding is well established and you are producing a good milk supply, your baby will never go off the breast while she is still getting an adequate amount from it to fill her up. You could give her an entire day's worth of bottles and she will always prefer the breast as soon as it is offered. Not one of the hundreds of babies I have worked with, or any of my three children have ever shown any reluctance to take the breast after a couple of bottle-feeds. In fact I tend to find the opposite happens with some babies. As your baby gets older – around six to eight weeks – they will become more and more established on the breast and can begin to refuse the bottle if it is not given on a daily basis. With some babies this is even more likely if they are given one bottle per day rather than two. My advice would be to do the 10:30 p.m. feed as a bottle initially, and then if you want to you can also change the night feed to a bottle of EBM, as described above.

- If you notice your baby does begin to fuss on the bottle and not really want to drink a lot, but will happily feed from the breast, then you have two options. You either continue with just one bottle-feed because you are not keen on the idea of doing a bottle-feed in the night, and hope things improve. In my experience this is usually the beginning of them refusing the bottle completely, and eventually she will not drink from it at all. As I said, a breastfed baby will always prefer the comfort of the breast, and after a short period of time you are likely to find that she just refuses the bottle completely.
- Your other option is to introduce a second bottle of EBM, either for the night feed, or as one of your day feeds. If you do a bottle for the night feed then use the methods described previously to get enough EBM for the bottle. Expressed milk is always the preferred option for the night feed, as it will be lighter on her tummy and not fill her up too much, which will make it easier to drop this feed when the time is right, giving

her a bigger appetite for her 7 a.m. feed. If you cannot produce enough milk to do the 10:30 p.m. feed and the night feed both as EBM, then any formula needed to supplement should be given at the 10:30 p.m. feed, rather than in the night. Infant formula takes longer for a baby's tummy to digest, so it can make them feel fuller for longer and not wake up as early as they would do after a breastfeed or bottle of EBM. This is only the case with some babies – others will sleep for the same period of time overnight whether they have had breast milk or formula. You won't know how it affects your baby unless you try it.

- If you would still prefer to do the night feed as a breastfeed then another option to introduce a second bottle is to give a bottle of EBM during the day. You can express your milk from the breast just before the time you are due to feed your baby and give it to her from the bottle instead. Your breasts will still continue to produce the milk for that feed because you are expressing it off and still telling your body that you need to make it. However, by giving it to your baby from the bottle, she will become a bit more used to drinking from it if she has begun to show signs that she would rather not.

CASE STUDY: Going back to work

Due to financial reasons I had to go back to work when my first baby was eight weeks old. I was working as a nanny and at the time the statutory full maternity pay only lasted 10 weeks, and we couldn't afford for me to take any extra time off. I was very lucky in that I only worked three days a week and my employer agreed to let my son come to work with me for one and a half days and my aunt, who was a registered childminder, agreed to look after him for the other one and a half days. I was still breastfeeding him and wanted to keep it up for as long as possible. He was already established on one bottle-feed per day (the 10:30 p.m.), but would never take very much at that time – usually 3–4fl oz (90–120ml) – but would still happily sleep through until around 4 a.m., when I would breastfeed him before putting him back to bed. I sent Jack off to my aunt's each week with enough expressed milk and bottles to last the entire day, which my aunt would feed to him. I would then express my milk at work at my son's regular feed times during the day to ensure I kept up my milk production. I would then store it in the fridge at work and bring it all home and freeze it that night.

My son proved very difficult for my aunt to feed for the first few weeks though. When the bottle of expressed milk was given to him each time, he really wasn't keen and would thrash around and cry. He would drink an ounce or two at most per feed to satisfy his immediate hunger but then get very upset if she tried to persevere and offer him any more. By the time I collected him at 6 p.m., he would be so hungry that he would spend the entire evening feeding to make up for him not being able to have the breast all day long! I remember one evening when I picked him up and he had literally just finished a bottle-feed. He had taken a decent amount for a change, as it was the end of the day and he was very hungry from snacking all day. I took him from my aunt to give him a cuddle and he immediately he started rooting around, head-butting me and trying desperately to get to the breast. I knew it wasn't because he was hungry because he had just finished a full bottle-feed. He merely wanted the comfort and reassurance of the breast after being apart from me all day – and wasn't going to settle down until I gave in!

My babies, like every other breastfed baby I've worked with, have always been well established on the breast before we offer them a daily bottle, so it doesn't cause any issues. It will only ever benefit you and your baby to get them used to a bottle from a young age. It will make life more practical at times, so that some pressure is taken off you, and other people can get involved with feeding and caring for your baby to give you some much-needed rest.

Ideally I would suggest introducing one to two bottles (whatever you have chosen and prefer) from around 14 days. This has always been the perfect age for every baby that I've worked with, as they are still young enough not to be fussy with the bottle. As soon as milk begins coming out of the teat, they will just drink it. Milk feeds hunger however it comes. It's only as they get older that they will begin to show a preference for the breast and will refuse the bottle. Many mums find this first introduction of the bottle as a little bit sad and want their baby to turn their nose up at the whole idea. 'Traitor' was my initial reaction the first time I watched all three of my babies drink their first bottle of expressed milk without a care in the world. Deep down, though, I was very pleased that they did drink it as it would give me another option if I needed to sleep and hand the rein to my husband.

If you are happy that your baby is established on the breast around day seven you can begin the bottle from then onwards. I have done this with some of the babies I have worked with who have been feeding well from the breast regularly without any fuss, and had no problems with them refusing the breast afterwards. My own daughter had a bottle of expressed milk at the age of five days, as my milk supply was a bit too much for her. She was also fine and happily went back on the breast at the next feed.

Although giving a baby a bottle makes sense from a practical point of view, some mothers still prefer to continue solely breastfeeding. That is absolutely fine too. If you are happy doing that, and don't have to worry about going back to work or being apart from your baby for any length of time, then you can continue to breastfeed solely for as long as you and your baby want to and as long as the milk supply is still there. Once you do stop, your baby can go straight on to having milk in a cup or beaker rather than a bottle if that's what you prefer. Details of which order to wean your baby's feeds are below.

Weaning off the breast

Weaning your baby off the breast is done using the same method of dropping feeds in a certain order, whether you plan to move her on to a formula feed to replace it, or need to drop the feed altogether because she has reached a certain age and no longer needs a particular feed.

Recommended weaning order

The order in which you should drop feeds are:

1: **3/4 a.m.** Night feed

2: **10:30 p.m.** This feed gets reduced and then dropped once your baby has been weaned. You should still continue to express at this time though to keep up your milk supply.

3: **10:30/11 a.m.** Replace this feed with a cup of water once protein has been introduced

4: **2:30 p.m.** This feed can be replaced with a cup of water or milk

5: **6/7 p.m.** To be replaced with a bottle or cup of milk before bed if under 2 years

6: **10 p.m.** Stop expressing using the breast pump at this time

7: **7/8 a.m.** Replace the morning feed with bottle or cup of milk if your baby is under 2 years

If you are weaning your baby off the breast because your milk supply has dwindled or you need to get her on to more bottles daily because you are going back to work, then using the recommended weaning order will work well. It means that you will still be able to breastfeed your baby for her morning and evening feed if that's what you would like to do. The easiest way to drop a feed is to give her a bottle for the feed you are dropping and just use the breast pump to lower your milk supply at that particular feed. Reduce the amount you pump off by 1fl oz (30ml) every three days until you are down to 1fl oz (30ml) from each breast. You can then drop the expressing altogether at that particular feed.

However, if you are dropping a feed because your baby has reached an age where she no longer needs it, but you do not need to give her a bottle as an alternative, e.g., the night feed, 10:30 p.m. feed or 11 a.m. feed, then you need to do things slightly differently. If she is currently breastfeeding at the feed that you are preparing to drop then you need to begin to reduce the amount of time she spends on the breast by five minutes every three days. Once she is down to a few minutes in total for her feed for three or more days in a row then you can drop the breastfeed altogether.

If you drop feeds in the order above then you shouldn't have any problems with your milk supply for the feeds that still remain, as your breasts will still be stimulated to produce milk at regular intervals during the day.

Dropping the night feed

The question every parent is desperate to know the answer to is: 'When will she drop her night feed and begin sleeping through the night?' The answer to this is simple: when you encourage and teach her how to wait a longer period of time by getting enough milk into her during the day, and teach her good sleeping habits from the start.

To start with, a baby will be unable to wait for a longer stretch of time in the night if she is not having enough milk between the hours of 7 a.m. and 7 p.m., even if she is having a late night top-up. There are certain key things you need to wait to happen before you can attempt to drop the night feed. These are:

- She is taking a minimum of 20–25fl oz (600–700ml) over a period of 24 hours, not including the night feed. If you are formula feeding this is easy to gauge. If you are breastfeeding then she should be feeding very well at all of her day feeds and taking a minimum of 4fl oz (120ml) expressed milk or formula in a bottle at the 10–11 p.m. feed.

- She is gaining a regular amount of weight each week – usually at least 3–5fl oz (90–150ml) – and your health visitor is happy.
- She is settling and sleeping well after the 10–11 p.m. feed, and not waking hungry until at least 3:30 a.m.
- She is settling well after the night feed and sleeping well until at least 7 a.m. without waking hungry before then. Babies come into a light sleep between 5 and 7 a.m. so it is very normal for them to be unsettled during that time of the morning without needing to feed. As long as she's not waking due to hunger then you can begin the process of dropping the night feed.
- You will probably begin to notice that she begins to want to take less at her 7:30 a.m. feed and doesn't seem as hungry and enthusiastic to finish this feed as she once was. She may even be taking less at the 10:30 a.m. feed too. This is a very big indicator that it is definitely time to begin watering down or reducing the night feed. Her appetite will then start to increase for her morning feeds again.

Please note

If you allow her to continue with the night feed and she carries on reducing her intake of milk at her two morning feeds, she will need to continue to feed at night to make up for the reduced amount of milk she is getting during her crucial day feeds. You then find yourself in a vicious circle, constantly trying to play catch up.

If you find that your baby is showing all of the above signs, then you can begin to reduce and drop the night feed altogether. In my experience I have found that most babies are ready to start this process around the age of five to six weeks. It is often a good idea to let her get over her six-week growth spurt before you begin to reduce her night feed.

If you feel that this is too early for your baby to drop her night feed, and you are happy to continue feeding her by breast or bottle in the night and would rather wait until she phases it out herself, that is fine too. Some babies will just gradually begin sleeping for longer and drop their night feed without too much fuss.

CASE STUDY

My two boys gradually slept for longer in the night and I began reducing the amount I gave them from the breast by a few minutes every few nights. They kept sleeping for longer and longer until finally they were going through to 7:30 a.m. by 12 weeks old.

Other more strong-willed babies will not sleep through without a bit more guidance. These babies will continue to wake for a night feed for as long as you offer it to them. There are even children who are still having two or three bottles or breastfeeds a night at the age of one to two years of age! All parents vary in what they are happy to do or not do with their baby.

Once you get to the stage where you feel that you are finally ready to encourage your baby to drop their night feed, and she's showing all of the signs listed, then it's best to use a gradual process over a period of weeks to get their tummy used to having a smaller amount, rather than forcing them to do it suddenly.

Below I have explained how to reduce the night feed whether your baby is bottle or breastfed and the gradual process and stages you should go through over a period of days and weeks, until you manage to drop the night feed altogether.

Reducing the night feed using a bottle

If your baby is currently taking a bottle of EBM or formula for her night feed and has been sleeping well at night, then you can begin to water it down. This involves putting less milk in the feed and adding some cooled boiled water, so that she is still having the same amount. I will work my example of how to reduce the feed in stages on the basis that your baby has been having a 4fl oz (120ml) bottle made up for the night feed. If she has been having a bigger one then you just need to alter the amount of scoops or water accordingly.

Watering your baby's feed down by making up the feed with less formula or adding water to breast milk is perfectly safe for your baby in the quantities I am suggesting for one feed per day. You do not need to worry about any adverse effects. I have worked with hundreds of babies, and have used this watering-down process with every single one of them, and haven't had any bad reactions. I believe it is the kindest way to encourage a baby to stop feeding at night. It allows their tummies to get used to the idea and go a longer stretch of time without needing to feed. She will then gradually begin to sleep for longer anyway and naturally push her wake-up time in the night to 5–5:30 a.m. once you begin the milk reduction.

You will find that the extra water does curb your baby's desire to feed during the night, but that is exactly what we are trying to encourage anyway. She will then increase the amount that she takes at the first morning feed, and even possibly the mid-morning feed too.

This watering-down process of encouraging your baby to drop the night feed only begins when you have already noticed that she is reducing one or two of her feeds by herself anyway. All you are doing is steering her in the right direction, by encouraging her to reduce and drop the night feed, rather than any of her day feeds.

I have heard some people recommend giving a baby sugar water when they wake in the night to encourage them to drop the night feed. This is because it is sweeter than just plain old water so a baby is more likely to drink it. Of course she will, but it will come at the expense of wrecking her new teeth. I am amazed that any health professional or carer would even suggest offering a baby sugar water anyway.

Formula bottle in the night

- You can water down this night feed by reducing the number of scoops that you put into your baby's bottle. Currently you should be adding four scoops of formula to 4oz (120ml) of boiled water. That is based on one scoop per 1fl oz (30ml) of water. When you begin watering down the feed then you still make up your usual 4fl oz (120ml) of water but instead of putting the full four scoops in as normal, then you should only put three scoops in to make up the feed.

- To start with, offer the formula feed with three scoops in to your baby when she wakes at her usual time in the night. Stick to this new consistency for a minimum of three nights or a maximum of seven. Once she is happily continuing to sleep until 7/7:30 a.m. before getting hungry and needing her morning feed, you can then make the second reduction.

- The next step is to put two scoops into 4fl oz (120ml) of boiled water. Again shake it up to mix the formula into the water, and feed it to your baby when she wakes for her night feed. It is a good idea to warm this feed slightly, even if you don't warm her other feeds. This is particularly important if it has been made up before you go to bed and is stored in the fridge. If it is warmed then she is much less likely to notice the thinner consistency of the milk with the reduced scoops, and drink it as if it is a full feed. Once she has been drinking this consistency and still happily sleeping until 7/7:30 a.m. before needing her next feed, then she will be ready for you to do the next drop down.

- You now need to make up 4fl oz (120ml) of boiled water and only put one scoop in it. With any luck, your baby should be sleeping well until 4–5 a.m. before waking now. It is this drop down that your baby is likely to notice, even if she didn't with the pervious drops in consistency. **I would still advise that you heat it before you give the feed to her. (Be aware that it will be taking less time to heat the more you water it down, as it is a thinner consistency.)**

- She may get a bit more frustrated as you offer her this new consistency, as she will be able to taste the difference. She may cry a little and pause as she's drinking it. Just persevere. Offer it to her, then if she cries take it out of her mouth and then offer it again.

- It's very normal for babies to not want to finish the full 4fl oz (120ml) at this stage, although some babies will still happily demolish the entire lot.

- If she has had a couple of ounces, then stop and wind her, and try to resettle her back to sleep rather than giving her the full feed. You may need to use the dummy for a few minutes if she's still unsettled and rooting around. Persevere with the dummy for a while. If she still refuses to settle, then offer her any of the feed that is still remaining and then try the resettling process with the dummy again. More often than not though, it is wind that is likely to be the cause of her refusing to go back to sleep.

Please note

Babies are always very unsettled and even possibly 'windy' during the 5–7 a.m. period in the morning up until the point you drop the night feed completely. Even if they have been sleeping soundly up until that point, giving the night feed and then trying to get them to go back to sleep again for another two to three hours is always very difficult. If you do manage to get her back in the basket after a night feed it is very normal for her to be in a very light sleep and need the odd pat or shhh to keep her settled until 7 a.m.

- After three to five days of this new consistency you may find that your baby naturally pushes her wake-up time to closer to 6 a.m. as her tummy gets used to not having a full feed. If she still continues to wake and drink the 4fl oz (120ml) with one scoop in, then it is time to drop down to just plain cooled boiled water with no formula added. As with previous bottles, heat it up and offer it to her when she wakes.

- Once you drop to just plain water **99** per cent of babies will decide that it's not worth waking for. You will most likely find that after two to three nights of offering her plain water she will begin to sleep better for the final couple of hours between 5 and 7 a.m. If she does wake then a pat or cuddle is usually enough to resettle her.

I've only had one baby out of all the hundreds I have worked with that still continued to wake and happily drink the full 4fl oz (120ml) cool boiled water. She was never any trouble – she would wake, drink the water and then go straight back down and sleep until we woke her between 7 and 7:30 a.m. We had to end up reducing her to 3fl oz (90ml) for three nights, then 2fl oz (60ml) and then she naturally began sleeping straight through without any fuss.

As she begins sleeping for longer at night and gets closer to the 7 a.m. feed anyway, your window of time of when to give the night feed reduces, regardless of the consistency stage. Coupled with the fact that you will be aware that as soon as you give it to her, then she is likely to be windy, and not settle back down as easily, you may be put off giving it to her at all.

I usually suggest that 5:30 a.m. is the latest time to offer a reduced night feed. If she wakes anytime after 5:30 a.m. and cries then I would suggest you try resettling her and encouraging her to wait for her 7 a.m. feed by using the following methods:

- Try not to pick her up, particularly if you are still breastfeeding during the day because she will smell the milk from your breasts, immediately start rooting around and be much harder to settle. Use the 'pat-and-shhh' technique as discussed on page 199 in Chapter 5, or rock the Moses basket to resettle her. You may have to do this on a few occasions over the following hour after she begins stirring to keep her settled to sleep until 7 a.m. This will help prevent her waking fully too early. If she is still rooting around as you do this then offer her the dummy and continue the pat-and-shhh technique while she remains in the basket. Five minutes of sucking on the dummy may be enough to resettle her properly without needing to feed her. You can then take the dummy away. Continue patting and shhing every now and again after you take the dummy away, and take these two comfort methods away slowly and one at a time, as discussed in Chapter 5.

- If patting and shhing doesn't work then pick her up and put her over your shoulder. Pat her back to check for wind initially. If she is okay, then just continue patting her bottom and saying 'shhh, shhh' to try to resettle her back to sleep.

- If you pick her up and she's rooting around and won't settle on you in the first couple of minutes of patting and shhing then offer her the dummy as you cuddle her. Continue with the pat-and-shhh technique as she sucks the dummy. If your baby is breastfed then picking her up at this time is very likely to cause her to root around for milk. You will have to be very strong to not give in. If she will not settle on you using the dummy, then another option is to ask your partner to try to resettle her. They will find it easier to settle her as they don't have the tempting breast milk smell. I always used to go in first and try to resettle at this time but more often than not it was my husband who took over, and would have a sleeping baby in his arms within five minutes flat.

- Once she's calm then try to put her back in her Moses basket/cot. You may need to continue patting for a few minutes, or allow her some extra time with the dummy when she first goes down, as she won't appreciate having all of her comfort taken away at once! If she wakes up then start the process from the top again, first settling in the basket, then moving on to the next steps and eventually picking up if she has woken right up again!

- Sometimes she will enjoy just lying next to you in the bed sleeping for the final hour before her 7 a.m. feed. It will keep her more settled while she is hungry and waiting that last stretch of time, and encourage her to continue sleeping up until the feed, rather than you battling with her in and out of the basket for the last hour. See the information on co-sleeping in Chapter 5 (page 203). If you are happy to do this then you will find she gradually stretches the period she sleeps overnight to closer to 7 a.m. anyway. A cuddle in bed first thing in the morning will not turn into a habit as long as this is the only time you do it at this age.

- Try to get her to wait to as close to her 7 a.m. feed time as possible. If by 6:30/6:45 a.m. you really can't stall her any longer, then I would advise on a split morning feed. Give her half of her formula feed or one breast, and then the other half around 7:30/7:45 a.m. If you were to give her the entire full feed at 6:30/6:45 a.m. she would then struggle to wait until the next planned feed time around 10:30/11 a.m.

- If, after trying the 'nice way' to resettle your baby when she wakes early each day, it just doesn't seem to be working then it may be wise to just put her back in her basket and let her have a little cry-it-out time. Try the above methods, but by 8–10 weeks she should have already mastered the art of being able to settle herself to sleep if you have been following a sleeping guide with her from an early age. If you know that she is able to settle herself for her day sleeps with a small amount of crying as she settles to sleep, then it is okay to try this if she continues to wake early every morning. With some strong-willed babies it is the only way to finally stop that early-morning waking. Go with your instincts. Usually babies just tend to sleep for longer and longer and finally make it to 7 a.m. without too much fuss. If yours doesn't seem to be stretching the time that she begins waking up and you have tried the above settling techniques, then leaving her to settle herself may be your only other option. Sometimes just putting her down and letting her cry for a few minutes means that she can get that initial anger out. Once she has got that out then she is more likely to respond and be comforted by a quick pat or shhh in the basket to help her drop right off to sleep. It really varies from baby to baby though, and in the eight to ten weeks since your baby has been born you will hopefully have learnt a few tricks on what works to help her settle.

CASE STUDY: Settling my babies

I had three very different babies. My first son was very good at settling himself from a very young age. He would cry very angrily for two to three minutes and then immediately stop, and seconds later he would be asleep holding his comfort blanket. As he got older and woke up because of illness or teething he would still always prefer to settle himself to sleep rather than be cuddled. I would go in if he woke crying in the night and check his nappy or put teething liquid on if I thought that was the problem. Once we had solved the problem, he preferred for me to just put him down and let him settle himself. He would usually cry for a few minutes but that was just his way of settling himself. If I tried to cuddle him back to sleep or pat or shhh him it would actually make him more unsettled and downright cross.

My second son was completely the opposite. If he begun crying we had to go to him immediately. If you didn't he would get more and more angry. I would pick him up to comfort him, then put him down (he'd still be awake but calm) and then just rest my hand on him. If he tried to get up or thrash around I would lay him back down. If he began crying a lot then I would pick him up over my shoulder and calm him down again. After a few attempts of this he would calm down and allow me to walk out of the room while he was half asleep. He is now almost seven and still needs to be talked out of a tantrum and calmed down with a cuddle. If he's left to his own devices he just gets himself more and more upset.

My daughter was different again. As a small baby she learnt to settle herself to sleep from around eight weeks onwards, with just a small amount of crying to get herself to sleep. As she got older she would still happily settle herself to sleep, sometimes with a bit of crying, but more often than not by singing herself to sleep. On the occasions where she has been teething or unwell then she loves nothing better than a cuddle to doze off in my lap. She then happily transfers to the cot. When she is well though, she will not entertain the idea of being cuddled to sleep. At

18 months she loves to have a book read to her, and then be put in her cot, zipped up in her grobag with her muslin to cuddle. We then wind her mobile up and she sings and chats until she drifts off to sleep. As long as we remember to do all of her 'bedtime ritual' then she settles just fine. If I were to try to put her down without a book, even for her lunchtime nap, she would create a big fuss and refuse to settle until I got her back up and read her the book!

All babies are different and you need to find what works for *your* baby. Only you will know what that is. I can only give you a guide of different things to try. Your job is to figure out which method your individual baby prefers, and helps her to settle.

If your baby continues to wake at 5 a.m. then you could also try pushing her late dream feed to 11 p.m. the previous night. I would only suggest this if your baby is happily sleeping between 7 and 10:30 p.m. and you have been waking her to do that feed. Pushing it to 11 p.m. will hopefully mean her early wake-up time will be pushed slightly later, maybe closer to 6 a.m. rather than 5 a.m. Do not be tempted to do the feed any later than 11 p.m. though. She will have already done a five-hour stretch between feeds from 6–11 p.m., and then you are asking her to do another one from 11:30 p.m.–7 a.m. If you push the 11 p.m. any later then you will be encouraging her long stretch to be at the beginning of the evening and night, rather than over the core night hours when you will need to be sleeping. Most parents are usually still up at 10/11 p.m. in the evening, so it makes sense to 'top-up' your baby at this time before you go to bed, in the hope that her long stretch of sleep will come when you need to be having yours.

Reducing an expressed breast milk (EBM) bottle in the night
This works in the same way as the formula in that you water it down, but you use expressed breast milk mixed with boiled water instead.

- Stage 1: Mix 3fl oz (90ml) EBM with 1fl oz (30ml) cool boiled water
- Stage 2: Mix 2fl oz (60ml) EBM with 2fl oz (60ml) cool boiled water
- Stage 3: Mix 1fl oz (30ml) EBM with 3fl oz (90ml) cool boiled water
- Stage 4: 4fl oz (120ml) plain cool boiled water.

Tip

Do not mix together until they are the same temperature. Let the boiled water cool down before mixing with the breast milk.

Use the above consistencies of expressed milk to boiled water, then use the same methods described above to wean your baby off her night feed.

Reducing and stopping a night feed if solely breastfeeding without the use of a bottle

If you have decided that you are happy to continue breastfeeding solely, without the use of a bottle, but want to know how to reduce and stop your baby breastfeeding at night then follow the steps below.

- The first thing I would suggest is that you read the feeding section and be sure that your baby is taking in enough breast milk during her day feeds. She needs to be drinking enough hind milk and be able to do a three-to-four-hour stretch between most of her day feeds before you can even consider conquering the night-time stretch. If she isn't able to do this, then she won't be ready to drop her night feed(s). Tackle your daytime routine first before you attempt to drop the night feed completely.

- Depending on how many times you are feeding your baby at night you can begin to reduce her milk intake between 11:30 p.m. and 7 a.m., which should then have the knock-on effect of increasing her appetite for her day feeds. Do this by reducing the time she spends on the breast by five minutes per feed every three nights. For example, if she's been having a 20-minute total feed time and then going back to sleep, then reduce this to 15 minutes. If she's unsettled and rooting around after the 15 minutes, then persevere with refraining from offering the breast again, and try to settle her with the dummy and cuddle.

- Continue to reduce the time spent on the breast by five minutes every three days. Once you are down to only five minutes spent on the breast then reduce down to a couple of minutes, and resettle with the dummy and cuddle. At this point having a husband or partner can come in very handy. It's a good idea to send them in now when the baby wakes because they will be more likely able to settle her with one of the methods listed earlier: pat, shhh; cuddle; dummy.

- It does take longer to convince a breastfeeding baby to drop the night feed but it is very possible with patience and perseverance!

CASE STUDY: Dropping the night feed of breastfed babies

My first two babies were breastfed in the night rather than bottle-fed. My eldest dropped his night feed at 14 weeks when he discovered his thumb! He had been doing pretty well anyway and going through until about 5:30 a.m., having a quick feed off one breast and then resettling until 7/7:30 a.m. Finding his thumb just gave him that extra bit of comfort to begin sleeping until 7 a.m. without a feed. My second son was 10 weeks when he dropped his night feed. Again, he had been going through until 5–6 a.m. and I was giving him a quick feed and then resettling him until the morning. With him I just gradually reduced the amount I was giving him, as described above.

My daughter had a bottle of EBM from the age of two weeks for her night feed, as well as EBM for her 10:30 p.m. feed. We began watering that feed down at just over six weeks, after she had her growth spurt, and by nine weeks she was no longer waking for it any more. If she woke on the odd occasion my husband would go in to resettle her so that she didn't smell the milk on me before the planned 7 a.m. feed.

Whichever method you decide to use to reduce and drop your baby's night feed is fine. It does have to be something you are both ready to do. Some parents are quite happy to continue feeding their baby in the night for as long as their baby wakes, and they hope that they will one day grow out of it and just stop waking. On the rare occasion this may happen, but be warned that the longer you continue night feeding the harder the habit becomes to break. As long as you and your baby are happy, that's all that matters and if you would prefer to continue then that is your prerogative.

Changes to milk feeds to coincide with weaning and getting older

Up until weaning age – around six months – your baby should continue on her same regular feed times that she started with from newborn. By the age of 10 weeks your baby should have settled into a good feeding routine if you have been trying to follow the guide times from the start. She should also have dropped her night feed or be well on the way to dropping it.

Recommended feed times for weaning
Before weaning on to solids begins, feed times are:

- *Between **7 and 8 a.m.***
- ***11 a.m.** Gradually push to this new time from the original 10:30 a.m. start that your baby needed in the early weeks*
- ***2:30 p.m.***
- ***6–6:15 p.m.***
- *Between **10 and 11 p.m.***

10:30 p.m. feed

If your baby is still waking in the night and seems genuinely hungry, then try to increase this feed by an ounce or two and also her day feeds as well. If she's bottle-fed then you may find putting her on a faster-flowing teat will not wear her out so much and she will be more likely to take a bigger feed at this time, which will then enable you to reduce and drop her night feed. If breastfeeding, then try to split the feed with a nappy change between breasts to wake her up a bit more again and get extra milk into her. You can also push the start time of the feed to 11 p.m. if your baby is still continuing to wake early each morning, as already discussed.

Some babies may start to take less at this feed than they do at all other day feeds. This is perfectly okay because this feed is purely a top-up, and babies will need varying amounts to get them through the night until their next feed at 7 a.m. The amount may also vary from day to day too, depending on how much milk she has taken during her day feeds between 7 a.m. and 7 p.m.

If your baby has only been drinking 2–3fl oz (60–90ml), or spending five minutes or less on the breast at this feed for more than three nights in a row, but still sleeping very well between 11 p.m. and 7 a.m. and is not waking hungry, then it is safe to drop this feed, even if you haven't already weaned her on to solids. I know many parents have been relieved to drop this feed as soon as possible after the night feed has been dropped, as they don't enjoy having to stay up late to do it.

However, you may find that your baby is happy to drop the 10:30 p.m. feed around 12–16 weeks, but you do run the risk, as she's gets closer to weaning age, that she may begin to wake in the night again because of hunger. If this happens then you need to reintroduce the 10:30 p.m. feed. Equally if she has only been drinking a small amount at this time she may need to have the feed increased as she gets closer to weaning age.

My personal preference is to keep the 10:30 p.m. feed as a 'safety net' until after you wean your baby on to solid food. Even if she is taking a reduced amount at that time it is my way of thinking that most parents, myself included, would prefer to do a feed at that time than drop it too early and run the risk of their baby waking up in the night hungry again. Once she has been weaned for two to four weeks and you feel that she is taking a good amount of solids at the 11 a.m. and 6 p.m. feeds, as well as an adequate amount of milk on a daily basis, then you can begin to reduce and drop the 10:30 p.m. feed.

How to drop the 10.30 p.m. feed

- To begin with, gradually bring it forward to a start time of 10 p.m. Start the feed 15 minutes earlier every fourth night until you have the feed starting at 10 p.m. As long as your baby is still sleeping happily through to 7 a.m. then you can begin reducing the amount.

- If you are bottle feeding reduce the amount you make by 1fl oz (30ml) every three nights, so on the fourth night drop down to the next lower mark on the bottle. Only make the reduction on the fourth night if your baby is still continuing to sleep well until 7 a.m. If you don't feel she's ready for the next reduction then stay at the amount you are giving for a few extra nights, and only make the reduction when you feel the time is right.

- If you are breastfeeding your baby for this feed then you can begin the reduction by giving her five minutes less as her total feed time every fourth night. Again, as with the bottle, only continue the reduction if your baby is still sleeping well between 11 p.m. and 7 a.m.

- Once she is down to 2fl oz (60ml) in a bottle or only five minutes on the breast at 10 p.m. for three nights or more, then you can safely stop the feed completely. Two fluid ounces (60ml) or five minutes on the breast is such a small amount of milk that, if she has been having that and still sleeping well, that amount will not be making a difference to how she is sleeping.

- It's important that when you start doing this milk reduction on the 10:30 p.m. feed that you do it as a dream feed (if you haven't already started doing that anyway), and try not to wake her too much. There will also be no need to change her nappy any more at this time (unless of course she's soiled), as that will encourage her to wake up a bit too much.

Top tip

Put two nappies on, one on top of the other, at 6 p.m. after you bathe her. Once you stop doing a nappy change at the 10:30 p.m. feed, her bedtime nappy needs to last 12–13 hours without being changed. That is a lot of wee to contain! I have found that boys in particular tend to produce a vast amount of wee, and are more likely to wake up wet through in the small hours and be difficult to settle back to sleep again if you have had to do a whole outfit and bed change!

It's important that you use a premium brand of nappy for overnight, even if you choose not to during the day to save a bit of money. The supermarket brands will almost certainly leak overnight as they are not designed to last for that length of time.

By adding the extra nappy you are just giving yourself and your baby some extra padding and an added safety net to ensure she doesn't wake up wet. The 'top' nappy can then be used first thing in the morning once you take the wet bottom nappy off, so you won't actually be wasting it or using any extra nappies.

7–8 a.m. feed

Before you drop the 10:30 p.m. feed you may find that your baby isn't as interested in this feed as she gets older, particularly once you begin weaning, which is another indicator that she is ready to drop that 10:30 p.m. feed. You may be waking her each morning and her enthusiasm may wane for this feed after the first initial few ounces or few minutes at the breast. Once you drop the

10:30 p.m. feed, her appetite for this feed should increase again. As long as you begin the feed by 8 a.m. at the latest, as your baby gets older and begins to sleep later in the mornings, then it won't have any effect on her next feed around 11 a.m.

11 a.m. feed

When you initially begin weaning, milk remains as the bulk of their feed at this time. It is only when protein and dairy are introduced some time later (see Chapter 6 for more details) that you can begin to reduce and drop this milk. Once your baby is happily taking a main meal containing some protein and then a pudding of either fruit/yoghurt etc., you can begin to reduce her milk intake at this time. Continue to give the milk before the solids, but reduce it using the same process suggested for the 10:30 p.m. feed by 1fl oz (30ml) or five minutes on the breast every three to four days. Once down to 2fl oz (60ml) or five minutes at the breast you can safely drop the feed altogether. This milk should be replaced with a cup of cool boiled water offered to your baby. Some parents prefer to give well-diluted baby juice in a cup. This is also an option but not necessary. As long as you persevere with the cup of boiled water she will begin to get more and more used to it and gradually increase her intake over a period of time. See Chapter 6 for more information on this too. As with everything, stick to the two Ps – patience and perseverance – and don't give up. My youngest still prefers water to juice at 18 months.

You will most likely find that your baby will increase the amount of solids she eats once this milk feed has been dropped, and will also increase the amount that she has been drinking at the 2:30 p.m. feed. As your baby gets older, you can gradually try to push this meal time closer to an 'official lunchtime' of 12 p.m., but this will largely depend on your baby's naps and how tired she is by lunchtime. I've always found that I can't get my babies to wait any longer than 11:15 a.m. if they haven't had a morning nap, otherwise they are just too tired to eat, and are generally falling asleep as they are eating their pudding!

2:30 p.m. feed

This milk feed will ideally continue until your baby is closer to one year old. It is something that most babies enjoy when they wake up from their lunchtime nap. If you find that she begins to reduce the amount that she wants to drink after her protein and pudding meal is introduced at lunchtime, then you could transfer this milk to a beaker or cup if you are bottle-feeding. (See Chapter 6, page 254, for advice on cups for milk.) If you are breastfeeding your baby during this feed you may find that she naturally reduces the amount she wants to take at this feed herself by spending less time on the breast.

Once you, or she, decide to drop this feed completely (which is usually by the age of 12 months), it can be replaced with a cup/beaker of water to drink when your baby wakes up from her lunchtime nap if you would prefer not to give her milk.

Tea. 6/6:30 p.m. milk feed

Between the ages of 7 and 12 months your baby's tea that initially is given with her milk feed around 6/6:30 p.m. will need to be moved to a separate time an hour or so earlier to help establish the three main meal times. How and when to do this is explained in more detail in Chapter 6, as well as what indicators will help guide you into knowing when to make the change.

Once you have established her tea at a separate time, you should be able to push her milk feed to between 6:30 and 7 p.m. for her to have before she goes to bed. This later time also enables her to build up more of an appetite for the milk, particularly after having her two-course meal an hour previously.

> ### One year old – tiered feeding times
> *At one year old your baby should be established on a tier method of feeding with milk and solids at different times:*
>
> | | |
> |---|---|
> | **7–8 a.m.** | Milk |
> | | Breakfast should be offered after morning milk |
> | **11–12 p.m.** | Lunch |
> | **2–3 p.m.** | Cup of milk or water |
> | **4:30–5 p.m.** | Tea |
> | **6:30–7 p.m.** | Milk |

At 12 months the guideline amount of milk that a baby should have as a minimum amount per day is between 10 and 12 fl oz (300–360ml), or two cups of milk. You can change her over to drink full fat cow's milk from 12 months, whether she has milk from a cup or still in a bottle for her morning and bedtime milk. If you are still breastfeeding you may prefer to just continue feeding her yourself for the two remaining feeds. As long as she is getting roughly this amount on a daily basis, made up from milk she drinks and also in the foods that she eats, then you can be sure that she is getting enough calories and nutrients she needs from her milk intake.

If she's teething or not very well at times then it is very normal for her to go off her food during these periods. Try not to worry – she will eat and drink when she's hungry or thirsty. All you can do is continue to offer her things and eventually her appetite will pick up again when she's feeling better, and probably even be slightly bigger for a few days to make up for the food she hasn't felt like eating while under the weather!

Sterilising can also be stopped completely at 12 months if you haven't already stopped.

5

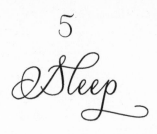

Sleep deprivation is about the only thing you can be certain of experiencing when you have a baby. No one will ever be able to explain how tough it is and nothing you have ever done before will ever quite prepare you for it. I've heard some people say that sleep deprivation has been used as a form of torture in some countries and that seems about right.

SIDS and sleep positions

The biggest subject surrounding babies sleeping is the worry of Sudden Infant Death Syndrome (SIDS). The original FSID (Foundation for the Study of Infant Death) charity has recently changed its name to The Lullaby Trust. The following information has been taken from their website:

'Sudden Infant Death' is the term used to describe the sudden and unexpected death of a baby or toddler that is initially unexplained. The usual medical term is 'sudden unexpected death in infancy' (SUDI). Some sudden and unexpected infant deaths can be explained by the post-mortem examination revealing, for example, an unforeseen infection or metabolic disorder. Deaths that remain unexplained after the post mortem are usually registered as 'sudden infant death syndrome' (SIDS)...

'Cot death' was a term commonly used in the past to describe the sudden and unexpected death of an infant. It has largely been abandoned, due to its misleading suggestions that sudden infant death can only occur when a baby is asleep in their own cot, which we know to be untrue.

What causes sudden infant death?

A thorough post-mortem examination will reveal a specific cause of death in less than half of all sudden infant deaths. Causes may include accidents, infection, congenital abnormality or metabolic disorder. For the deaths that remain unexplained (SIDS), researchers think there are likely to be undiscovered causes. For many it is likely that a combination of factors affect a baby at a vulnerable stage of development.

Over 300 babies still die every year of SIDS in the UK. Research has shown that several maternal and infant care factors are more frequently associated with babies who die of SIDS, than with those that survive. While it is clear that not all the factors are modifiable, there are some that are amenable to change in order to reduce the risk of SIDS. As such, The Lullaby Trust, along with many other organisations, provides advice for parents to reduce the risk of SIDS.

While SIDS is rare, it can still happen and there are steps parents can take to reduce the chance of this tragedy occurring. This guide lists the essential things you can do or avoid doing, to help lower the chance of SIDS. You can also talk to your midwife or health visitor if you have any concerns or contact The Lullaby Trust directly.

- Place your baby on her back to sleep (not front or side)
- Keep your baby smoke free during pregnancy and after birth
- It is safest for your baby to sleep in a crib or cot in the same room as you for the first six months, even during the day
- Use a firm, flat, waterproof mattress in good condition
- Don't cover your baby's face or head while sleeping or use loose bedding
- Do not let her get too hot. Keep her head uncovered
- Place your baby with her feet to the foot of the cot, to prevent her wriggling down under the covers
- Don't sleep with her on a sofa or armchair – sofa sharing with your baby greatly increases the chance of SIDS
- Breastfeed your baby
- Settle to sleep (day and night) with a dummy. This can reduce the risk of cot death even if the dummy falls out while she sleeps. Encouraging her

to suck as she gets sleepy means she is likely to continue making the sucking movement even after the dummy has been taken away

It is dangerous for your baby to sleep in your bed if you (or your partner) smoke, drink or take drugs:

- *Bed-sharing increases the chance of SIDS and is particularly dangerous if either you or your partner smokes (even if you do not smoke in the bedroom or anywhere else at home)*
- *If you or your partner have drunk alcohol or taken drugs (including medication that may make you drowsy)*

Also:
- *If your baby was premature (born before 37 weeks)*
- *Is less than four months old*
- *If your baby weighed less than ½lb (2.5kg) at birth.*

In doing or complying with all of the above, which is all taken from The Lullaby Trust website, it is thought that your baby will have a lower chance of being affected by SIDS.

With my children I complied with these guidelines with the exception of two points, and this was clearly my own personal decision. Firstly, all of my children moved from our room to the nursery by the age of 10 weeks, which was my personal preference. As previously described, I had an Angelcare movement mat in my baby's cot, which monitored their breathing and would have alerted me on the parent unit in my bedroom if there had been a problem. For me personally, this gave me the reassurance and confidence to move my baby to a separate bedroom. It may not be the case for all parents and if you prefer to keep your baby in your room with you for the first six months, as per The Lullaby Trust guidelines, this is absolutely what they would recommend and I would never advise against it.

Secondly, I also decided against using the advised sleeping position of putting a baby to sleep on her back.

Again this was my own personal choice and based on what I did with my first baby 10 years ago. At that time the SIDS guidelines were to place a baby to sleep on their side with rolled-up towels or blankets behind and in front of them, to wedge them firmly in and prevent them rolling on to their front or back by accident. You could then place a thin sheet or even muslin over the top of them and tuck it down the sides of the blankets or towels to keep them in position. At the time, the thinking was that tummy sleeping was unsafe for a newborn because they cannot lift their head, so are in danger of suffocating.

Laying a baby on their back to sleep was also deemed less safe in case a baby should vomit and choke. It was suggested that when a baby was sleeping on their side any vomit or mucus would just trickle out of their mouth, rather than cause them to choke.

I used this advice for my firstborn and it worked well for him. He was a C-section baby and was full of mucus from the birth (see feeding section page 101 for more info on this) and was comfortable in this position. Once he had cleared the mucus I found he really enjoyed sleeping this way. In my opinion, it was a much more like the natural foetal position that he was already used to from being in the womb. I continued to always put him to sleep on his side with rolled-up towels either side in his Moses basket. Being a big baby he moved to his cot at six weeks, as he no longer fitted in his basket comfortably. I did the same with the rolled-up towels in his big cot too. Once he began rolling from side to side, around the age of four to five months, I removed the towels. As soon as he learned to roll on to his tummy that was always then his preferred sleeping position. I always put him down on his side, but would inevitably find him on his tummy with his bottom sticking up in the air when I went to check on him.

My second baby was born in 2006 and I hadn't realised that the recommended sleeping position for babies had changed. Having had another C-section, I had another baby full of mucus and it was only natural and instinctive for me to put him on his side to sleep, as I knew that it had worked well for his brother. Because The Lullaby Trust guidelines had changed since I had my first baby, the hospital naturally wanted to lie my son on his back to comply with the new guidelines. Unfortunately, because he had so much mucus he kept on choking and having difficulty breathing.

I had restricted movement due to my operation so I felt it was even more essential to lie him on his side as I wouldn't be able to get to him quickly if he was struggling.

In the end I took the decision that he would be more comfortable sleeping on his side like his elder brother. He was a very sicky baby, always vomiting after a feed, so I felt that it was even more crucial to lie him on his side to sleep. By having him lie on his side to sleep, even if he was sick while lying in his basket/cot at night after a feed (which he often was), it would just trickle out of his mouth and land on the muslin that I had stretched over his Moses basket sheet. He would carry on sleeping and I would change the muslin whenever he had vomited on it and place a fresh one under his head. We didn't have any more choking incidences with him lying on his side, and once he began moving around in his big cot, I again removed the rolled-up towels, and he was a tummy sleeper just like his big brother as soon as he learned to roll over.

In my experience a baby doesn't turn their head to the side to allow any mucus or vomit to come out. Their natural reaction is to panic because the vomit affects their normal breathing rhythm.

My daughter was also fairly sicky at times, so this sleeping position also helped her. I did observe on countless occasions as I laid her on her back just to change her nappy that she would still panic and need picking up if she began to vomit while I was changing her. All this would be while she was wide-awake and happened frequently up until the age of six to eight months.

Side-sleeping was my personal choice and I am not recommending to parents that they go against The Lullaby Trust guidelines. However, side sleeping with towels is an option you could explore with a healthcare professional if your baby is very sicky, or has a lot of mucus, wind or reflux.

In my experience some babies like mine can sleep better when placed on their side with the rolled-up blankets/towels for a number of reasons:

- The rolled-up towels make her feel cuddled and snug in her basket/cot
- It is a more natural foetal position
- It is a more comfortable position for a baby who struggles with excess wind, colic or reflux
- If she were to vomit it would just trickle out of her mouth on to the muslin
- It is a better position if she has a cold or blocked nose, to be able to breathe better. You can also place a blanket or towel underneath the mattress at the head end to prop up if needed. This helps to alleviate pain that a reflux or very windy baby may experience, or help a baby with a cough or cold breathe more easily

If you and your healthcare professional decide that your baby might benefit from sleeping on her side then lie her on the right side rather than her left. This is because the tummy is on the left side of the body so I have found that babies are more likely to be sick if put on this side immediately after a feed. It is also important to put her in so that her feet are at the very bottom of the Moses basket or cot, to prevent her slipping under any blankets you place over her. Wedging her in between the rolled-up towels or blankets tightly should prevent this, but it's always good to be thorough.

The picture opposite shows you exactly how to position the towels in the Moses basket to ensure that your baby is safe and will not roll on to her front. Hand towels or cellular blankets are the best things to roll up and place one in front of her and one behind her. The towels should only come as high as your baby's armpits, as pictured, so that her face is completely uncovered.

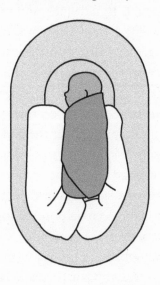

In my opinion the idea to place some babies on their side to sleep has many benefits, all of which allow you and her a more restful sleep.

Once a baby is of an age where she can roll from front to back and back to front she may prefer to sleep on her tummy. As this usually happens once a baby is over four months anyway, it is okay to allow her to do this. By this age her head and neck control should be very good, so there will be less likelihood of her suffocating, which is the reason tummy sleeping is discouraged in small babies. Always put her down to sleep on her side or back, but if you go in to check her once asleep and she has rolled herself on to her tummy and is sleeping happily then try not to worry. You can buy a movement mat to monitor her breathing if you are really worried about this. Once a baby finds a preferred position of sleeping on their tummy, there isn't anything you can do to change it, but the movement mat that 'keeps a check' on her breathing will give you some reassurance.

Many of the mothers that I have worked with have tried their baby in the side position and continued with it, noticing a big difference in their baby's sleep. Some mums have preferred to stick to lying their babies on their back to sleep, which is absolutely fine and in line with the current guidelines, and their baby sleeps well in that position. Equally, I have also worked for a few mothers who insist on placing their babies on their tummies to sleep, as they have found that worked with previous children – although this isn't something I would recommend for a newborn baby. Always try to encourage your baby to sleep on their back when you first bring them home from hospital, as per the NHS and Lullaby Trust guidelines. The alternative side sleeping position has been suggested as an alternative that worked for me and many other mums, because our babies had problems that lying on their backs added to (see page 160). My method for sleeping position for a baby with health difficulties, like reflux or excess sickness after feeds, is different from the advice for sleeping a baby to protect against SIDS. If you are unsure then you can speak to your paediatrician, doctor or health visitor before making any decisions where a complex risk assessment is being undertaken (e.g., reflux vs SIDS).

As a parent it is your choice to lay your baby in the position you are most comfortable with. However, please read all of the information from the NHS and The Lullaby Trust website and also listen to advice from other parents. You need to make a decision after weighing up various risk factors and take into account the individuality of your particular baby. Bear in mind that the sleeping position that worked for your first baby may not work for your second. Trust your instincts and do what you feel is right.

Swaddling your baby

Many babies also enjoy the feeling of being swaddled in the early weeks. The comfort of being wrapped up tightly helps them to sleep more soundly and for longer periods.

Follow the steps in the illustration below to swaddle your baby. It needs to be done quite tightly as many babies would give Houdini a run for his money! If they do manage to get out of

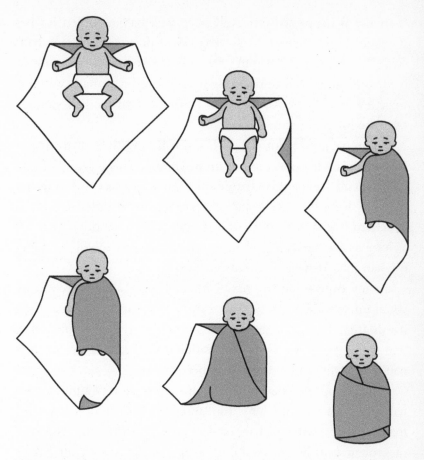

their swaddle they can become very unsettled until reswaddled again, and you don't want to end up having to do this repeatedly in the middle of the night. You need to ensure that the swaddle is quite tight around the top half of her body but make sure her hips and legs are NOT swaddled too tightly as she needs to have free movement in her legs. It becomes much easier the more you do it.

Swaddling is a great idea up to the age of around six weeks. At this age you can begin to try half-swaddling your baby for her daytime sleeps. Follow the steps pictured but leave her arms out. Once you begin half-swaddling I would advise you give your baby a muslin square to cuddle. This gives her something to do with her 'new found arms' that she hasn't been used to having out while sleeping.

If she is happy to settle and sleep well half-swaddled for her daytime sleeps, then you can progress to putting her down half-swaddled for her 7–10 p.m. sleep. If she is then continuing to settle and sleep well during this sleep while being half-swaddled for a few days in a row, then you continue with the half-swaddle over the full night-time period.

Some babies do not cope well with having their arms free at this age, even if given the muslin to cuddle. This is why I always recommend trying this change on a gradual process during her daytime sleeps first. If she still prefers to sleep swaddled and is too unsettled half-swaddled, then it is fine to keep swaddling her for as long as she needs it. I've known some parents to still be doing it when their baby is six months or more.

In my experience the reason that babies wake up frequently when un-swaddled (particularly boys), is because as soon as their hands are free, they begin to suck on them, and the stimulation of that wakes them up. In being swaddled they cannot get to their hands so easily, and tend to sleep better.

Another option you can try if you want to stop swaddling your baby, but are finding she is too unsettled with having her arms free, is to use a baby grobag, or sleeping bag, with arms. This type of grobag usually has very long arms, which cover your baby's hands, so, although she won't be swaddled, she also won't be able to get to her hands to suck them and become unsettled. Obviously this is a bit more difficult if it is summertime and the weather is hot, although you could then reduce the numbers of layers that she is wearing under the bag.

Developing sleep routines

Newborn babies tend to sleep a great deal in the first few days and weeks after birth. This is very normal. They may wake up slightly to 'ask' for a feed, or during nappy changes, but usually want to go back to sleep very quickly once the feed is over – and, in the case of a breastfed baby, fall asleep as she is feeding or at the end.

Parents are often lulled into a false sense of security, boasting to friends and family that they have a baby who feeds and sleeps wonderfully all the time. In truth, all babies are very good sleepers in the first couple of weeks after birth. They also have the potential to continue being good at sleeping if they are taught the correct sleep associations from a very young age, and not left to develop bad sleeping habits over time. Babies learn what you teach them. Only you as the parent can guide your baby towards good sleeping habits.

Many parents that I have worked with say that their baby started off being a good sleeper but then it all went wrong. It can sometimes coincide with an illness or going away on holiday, where your baby's normal routine has been broken to fit in with your plans. It is fine to do this in the short term if you go away for a couple of nights. Being somewhere different can mean you have to put your baby to bed at varying times. Even if you try to stick to your usual routine and get her to bed on time, she may be so unsettled in her new environment that you have to settle her in a different way.

My sons would settle and sleep anywhere and not be phased by new environments. My daughter, however, is very different; she settles herself from awake and sleeps wonderfully at home in her own cot but becomes very unsettled and upset if we have to get her to sleep anywhere else, like her grandparents' or hotels while on holiday. If my parents are looking after her overnight, then my father usually lets her fall asleep in his arms at a later-than-normal bedtime and then transfers her to the cot. If they try and put her into the cot awake to go to sleep she goes ballistic and screams until she makes herself hoarse. They have found a routine that works for them, and when she comes home she settles as usual in her own cot by herself. We went on holiday when she was 12 months and she was the same in the travel cot there. I used to walk her round in the pushchair until she fell asleep and then transfer her to the travel cot where she would sleep all night. If she stirred or cried then a quick pat and reassuring shhh from me to let her know I was there would settle her again. As soon as we returned home we resumed our normal routine of putting her in the cot awake and she was absolutely fine and settled herself without a problem.

While away from the usual home environment you just have to do what works at times to enable you all to get a good night's sleep. The crucial thing to remember is that once home you need to go back to your baby's normal routine as quickly as possible. She may be unsettled at times over the first 24 hours, particularly if she is exhausted from being away from home and having had less sleep. She may also initially 'test' you to see if she can get you to continue with any bad habits that may have been created. As long as you are consistent she will quickly settle down.

Illness can also throw a spanner in the works of any routine. If your baby is unwell it is usually best to just 'go with the flow.' Attempt to follow your daily feed and sleep times but you mainly just need to trust your instincts and do what you feel is right. If she's unwell she will most likely need to sleep more and for longer anyway – sleep is the best cure for most illnesses and helps the body to fight off infection and get well again. (Although being too sleepy and lethargic is not a good sign and you should take your baby to see a doctor if you are worried.)

She may not feel hungry or want to take any milk or solids at the usual times. However if she then shows signs of hunger an hour or two later, then you need to let her feed. If your baby is already at an age where she has dropped her 10:30 p.m. feed, as well as her night feed, then you can reintroduce it as a one-off if you feel that she has not eaten enough during the day to be able to last all night. It is much better to offer an extra feed in the evening than to go down the route of giving her a feed in the middle of the night once she has already dropped that feed.

Once you have dropped the night feed, I wouldn't recommend ever giving in and allowing her any milk during the core night hours between 11 p.m. and 7 a.m. again. You can always have a bottle or cup of cool boiled water prepared just in case you were to need something. If she is genuinely thirsty in the night then she will happily take some of this anyway.

Offering a night feed even as a one-off can be risky, as your baby can slip back into the habit of waking in the night expecting to get it again on subsequent nights. Once you have given in once, it is much more likely you will relent a second and third time, and, before you know it, you will be back to a regular night waking with your baby always expecting to be fed.

Bad sleep associations don't just crop up when babies are ill or on holiday. Many books and health professionals encourage parents to feed their baby on demand. This leads to mothers offering milk to their baby every time she wakes and roots around. The rooting reflex is a perfectly normal newborn reflex and one which they display almost as soon as they wake anyway, although it doesn't always mean a baby needs to be fed immediately. With some perseverance you can usually delay the feed for a while, which will encourage her to take a bigger feed later. If a baby is fed every time she wakes, then she is likely to turn into a snack feeder, which can lead to terrible problems with wind or – worse – colic and reflux, which will affect her ability to sleep well.

Breastfeeding mothers are told that if they demand feed their baby she will eventually find her own sleep routine and settle down with time. Although a very small minority of babies may do this (nothing is impossible), most babies will not, and will still be feeding two to three times or more over the core night period at the age of six months. This continues until the parents are so exhausted they ask for help.

In reality, most babies who are demand fed spend less than half the amount of time on the breast at each feed than a baby in a three-to-four-hourly feeding routine would. This means that a lot of the milk that they are drinking will be mostly fore milk and not the important hind milk.

The fore milk can be compared to a 'starter' in a restaurant. It whets your appetite but it is never going to sustain you for a decent period of time. Understandably, snacking on fore milk is never going to sustain your baby for a three-to-four-hour stretch between feeds. (See Chapter 4, page 65, for more info on this.) Therefore your baby will wake again one to two hours later looking for more milk and is likely to just want to snack feed again, because she hasn't built up a big enough appetite to need more.

Equally formula-fed babies who demand fed may only take a very small feed and then look to be fed a couple of hours later. This snack feeding on demand leads to a vicious circle of the baby waking constantly, day and night, to be fed. A newborn baby is able to manage one longer stretch of between four and six hours without a feed per 24 hours if she is mostly fed every three to four hours. The time you would try to plan this stretch is over the core night period between 11 p.m. and 4 a.m. The longest stretch that you will get from a baby that is being demand fed during the day every one to two hours is a three-to-four-hour gap from one feed to the next, although it is more likely that she would rather continue waking frequently at night to snack!

Parents continue with this demand feeding day and night and, by the time their baby is three to four months old, have usually reached breaking point with exhaustion. They realise that nothing seems to be changing, their baby is not settling themselves into a routine as predicted, and they have now resorted to rocking, patting and feeding their baby to sleep to get them to settle. For some parents the breaking point comes later, but it usually comes eventually: that point where you are so sleep deprived that you realise that, unless you do something to change the bad sleep habits your baby now has, you will have to continue with no end in sight.

If your baby has developed bad sleep associations they can be corrected. The younger the baby, the easier it is to encourage a better sleep routine, but it is still possible to turn things around if your child has reached the age of two or three. I have consulted with three different sets of parents with two-year-olds who are waking repeatedly at night, and being brought into their parents' bed to sleep. I have given them clear instructions on how to break the bad habits formed and get their children sleeping better and in their own bed. Within a week their children were no longer coming into their parents' beds, and were settling and sleeping in their own beds all night. I never even had to meet the parents or child as the consultations and follow-up were all done on the telephone. If you are prepared to put in the hard work in establishing a routine then everyone is so much happier.

I believe it's so important to do this from a young age. If you teach your baby how to 'settle herself' from an early age then you will never have the problem of bad habits developing.

It is not 'luck of the draw', as some parents suggest, as to whether you get a baby who is a 'good sleeper' or 'bad sleeper'. *All* babies have the potential to continue being 'good sleepers' after that initial two-week post-birth sleepy phase. It is up to you as her parents to encourage and teach her the correct sleep associations with consistency, patience and perseverance! This will ensure she remains able to continue sleeping well throughout her childhood. How we sleep is based, in large part, on habit and what our bodies use as the signals that it is time to sleep. The things that you teach her and encourage her towards in the first year of her life will set her up in good stead for the rest of her childhood.

When can I start a sleep routine?

As long as you begin your feeding routine when you come home from hospital and are ensuring that she is getting good-quality feeds on a regular basis, then your baby should be settling and sleeping very well between feeds for the first couple of weeks at least. It is very normal for a newborn baby to sleep for as much as 16 hours a day (or even more), often in stretches of three to four hours at a time. Like the sleep all of us experience, babies too go through different stages of sleep: drowsiness, REM (rapid eye movement) sleep, light sleep, deep sleep and very deep sleep. A newborn may wake to ask for a feed and have their nappy changed, but usually will fall asleep during the feed or within half an hour after it. Let her sleep as much as she wants to between three-and-four-hourly feeds in the daytime for the first couple of weeks. It is very unlikely to have any impact on your nights in making her more wakeful.

Once your baby is able to stay awake for one and a half hours then you can begin to implement the sleep routine effectively. This usually happens between the ages of two and four weeks, but varies from baby to baby.

Beginning to implement the sleep routine

More than anything, once you implement a sleep routine, it is very important that you keep track of the last time that your baby woke up. This is because a very young baby has a breaking point where they can tip over into the realm of being overtired after a certain length of time awake. An overtired baby will be almost impossible to settle for hours on end, no matter what you try. Eventually they will just pass out through sheer exhaustion. However, they are more likely then to sleep fitfully and wake frequently.

A parent who says their baby cries all evening, won't go to sleep, and has been diagnosed by their doctor as having colic, could just have a baby that is becoming overtired each evening. Babies who are overtired will cry incessantly. Nothing you do will seem to settle them, and, even through they may drift in and out of sleep, they will continue to wake up again and resume their wailing. Many parents assume their baby must be in some sort of pain, and, when they describe what is happening to their doctor, colic is diagnosed. This overtiredness is more likely to happen at the end of the day and go on into the evening, just as colic is usually more likely to happen in the evenings. Eventually the final thing that settles the baby is usually allowing her to become hungry enough to take her 10:30 p.m. feed. This usually makes her feel so full and sleepy that she will finally settle down as she is so exhausted from being awake for hours.

Out of all the hundreds of babies I have worked with, only one has genuinely suffered from colic and reflux connected to food allergy or intolerance (see case study, page 110, in the feeding section). It is my belief that, if you implement a feeding and sleep routine from a young age, then your baby has no need to cry continuously for long periods of time. All of her physical needs are being met through being encouraged to feed regularly and she will be encouraged to sleep at times that work well with her body's natural sleep rhythms. Babies don't need to be so unhappy and I would be very worried if any of the babies I worked with were crying incessantly for long periods of time. Of course, babies cry, for varying reasons that are explained later on, but continuous crying that cannot be appeased is always a concern. If your baby is following the feeding and sleep guide that I have suggested, but still crying for long bursts, then it is well worth seeing your GP to rule out any medical problem.

The crucial time-window rule is two hours. This is the absolute maximum time a young baby up to the age of around eight weeks is able to stay awake before becoming overtired. This means that once your baby has been awake for one and a half hours, you need to begin 'winding her down' so that she can become sleepy enough to be completely asleep and settled by the two-hour mark. If you miss that window for some reason, it is very possible that you will have a grouchy, irritable crying baby for the next hour or two (at least).

Most babies do not generally show signs of beginning to get tired when they are very young. They can be fine one minute and very quickly start crying and refusing to settle. This usually happens when they have gone past the two-hour window of awake time. I have heard it said by so many people, 'She never looks tired, so I don't put her down for naps.'

Quite often, babies are just left to doze as and when, as parents are unsure what is a normal amount of sleep for a baby to have. Up to the age of 10 weeks it is quite normal and healthy for a baby to be sleeping for around 16 hours in any 24-hour period. This is made up of between four and six hours of sleep between 7 a.m. and 7 p.m. and then also sleeping in the evening and night. Babies who are encouraged into a sleep routine from a young age develop a much better ability to sleep well throughout babyhood and childhood.

A baby who is left to find their own sleep routine and only ever doze off in a pushchair, car seat and on a play mat is very likely to be much more unsettled during the day and night. She will be irritable even when awake during the day because she isn't getting any quality sleep in a quiet environment.

All babies come into a light sleep 30–60 minutes after they have drifted off to sleep. It is at this point that they will either wake up or drift into a deeper sleep. If your baby is taught the correct sleep associations from a young age and learns how to settle herself, then she is much less likely to wake herself up as she drifts between the stages of sleep, and will then drop into a deeper sleep.

The four stages of sleep

1: *Drowsiness: the eyes droop and may open and close as she dozes.*

2: *Light sleep: she moves and may startle or jump when she hears noise.*

3: *Deep sleep: in deep sleep your baby will breathe deeply and regularly, sometimes with a big sigh. She will lie still but may move her arms or legs and move a little and make little sucking movements with her mouth or suddenly give a start. These sudden movements of the whole body are called hypnagogic startles and are perfectly normal. I'm sure you may have even experienced them yourself as you drift off to sleep.*

4: *Very deep sleep: quiet and the baby doesn't move.*

The usual cycle of sleep is stage 1 at the beginning of the sleep cycle and then stage 2, then 3, then 4. She will then move back to stage 3, then 2 and then to REM sleep.

REM (rapid eye movement) sleep is a lighter sleep when dreams occur and the eyes move rapidly back and forth. Although babies spend around 16 hours a day sleeping, about half of this is in REM sleep. Older children and adults sleep fewer hours and spend much less time in REM sleep.

The above cycles may occur several times during sleep. Babies may awaken as they pass from deep sleep to light sleep in the first few months and may have difficulty going back to sleep if they are taught the wrong sleep associations.

A baby who is not 'put down' to sleep in a quiet environment for her day as well as night-time sleep is highly likely to wake when she drifts into a light sleep. This can then lead to her only ever 'cat-napping' during the day, where she just has short sleeps of between 30 and 60 minutes. If a baby is never taught or encouraged to settle into a deeper sleep at least once during the day, how can she be expected to be able to do it at night-time? She will continue naturally to wake up during the night every time she drifts into that light sleep, and then expect you to help her get back to sleep as she doesn't know how to do it on her own.

Research has proven that all babies drift into a light sleep repeatedly during the night, just as we as adults do. It is only the babies who are taught the wrong sleep associations who are unable to resettle themselves.

The sleep routine that I have used for all three of my children, and the one that I give the mothers I work for as a guideline, ensures that your baby goes down for her naps before she becomes overtired. I believe that it is very important to put your baby in a quiet, dark environment during her daytime naps as well as her night-time sleep. Ideally the nursery would be the best place if you are at home, but a pushchair or pram that lies flat, or a travel cot in a dark room at a friend or relative's house will also be fine.

I have heard so many people say, 'Oh your baby must have her day and night round the wrong way,' about babies that are unsettled and wakeful at night.

The aim is to distinguish between sleep and awake time *not* day and night.

Sleep is a quiet, dark place away from noise and stimulation, where a baby can enjoy quality sleep.

Awake is a light, airy environment with noise and stimulation, so that she understands it is playtime.

If you do this, and structure your baby's sleep, then you won't have any problems with your baby being more wakeful during the night in particular.

Although it is good for a baby to get used to hearing noises as they sleep and not be disturbed by it, that is totally different to being expected to just doze off and have a good sleep right in the middle of the family home, with everything going on around her. Would you enjoy a quality sleep in the middle of the living-room floor while the TV was on, people were in and out of the room and the curtains were wide open with sunlight streaming in? I think each of us would have the same answer to that question!

The sleep routine below can be used as soon as your baby shows that she is able to stay awake for around one and a half hours after a feed, which generally happens between the ages of two and four weeks. This sleep routine should be used as a guide only. Babies need varying amounts of sleep. Some may need to go to sleep 10–15 minutes earlier or later than the times stated and other babies will wake up earlier than the time stated or some may even need to be woken up. You need to establish what works for your baby. As your baby gets older the naptimes will need to be adjusted accordingly. How and when to do this is explained below.

> **Sleep routine**
> **Wake** 7–8 a.m.
> **Sleep** 8:30 –10:15 a.m.
> **Sleep** 11:40 a.m.– 2:15/2:30 p.m.
> **Sleep** 4–5:30 p.m.
> **Sleep** 6:45 p.m.–10/10:30 p.m.
> **Sleep** 11 p.m. – 7 a.m. (with night feed somewhere during this time)

You can use the next sleep that your baby is due to have as your indicator as to whether she has had enough or too much sleep at the previous naptime. The lunchtime sleep is the longest one and will be the nap that continues until your baby is between 18 months and 3 years (or longer for some children), even after the other naps have been dropped.

The above sleep times fit in with all of the feed times already discussed in Chapter 4. The feed times are included below for ease of reference. The aim is your whole day should flow from one thing to the next, making life less stressful for you and your baby.

Getting up
In my experience babies that are encouraged and allowed to sleep in until 7:30 a.m. are happier, and find it easier to make it through to the next naptime without dozing off. I have also found that if you encourage this habit from a very early age you are much more likely to have a baby who continues to sleep until well after 7 a.m. naturally as she gets older, rather than regularly waking at 6 or 6:30 a.m. to start her day.

7/8 a.m. breast- or bottle-feed
Wake her at 7:30 a.m. if she is still sleeping and do your morning breast- or bottle-feed. A nappy change or face wash around 8:15 a.m. is usually enough to stop her dozing off too early if she is looking sleepy.

If she wakes earlier than 7 a.m. to try and encourage her to doze off again until it gets closer to 7 a.m. Sometimes a cuddle in bed with you will work. Depending on what time she fed in the night she may be genuinely hungry. You can offer her half of her full breastfeed if she is awake due to hunger, which will probably make her doze back off again. The earliest I would advise beginning a split feed on a baby that is wide-awake and refusing to go back to sleep is 6:45 a.m. Give her one breast or half of her normal bottle-feed and try to encourage her to doze back off until around 7:45 a.m. At this point you should wake her. The feed can then be finished by offering her the second breast or the remainder of a formula feed. It is important that she has completely finished feeding by 8:15 a.m. in order not to take her hunger away for the next feed. If she has had a split feed and had to be woken again at 7:45 a.m. then she should be ready to go down for her morning nap somewhere between 9 and 9:30 a.m., and sleep until around 10 or 10:15 a.m. Remember to stick to the two-hour sleep rule in the first eight weeks.

If she has been wide-awake from 7 a.m. or earlier and refused to go back to sleep despite a split feed, then she will be very tired before the usual start time of the morning nap. Try to keep her awake for as long as possible to get as close to the naptime as you can, but do not allow her to break the two-hour rule of awake time. Roughly one and a half hours after she woke she will begin to get sleepy. Wind her down by making sure she is in a quiet, dark environment and ready to sleep, then put her down. If you have a school or nursery run to do then she can have this nap in the car seat or pushchair. If she has woken early then she will need the extra sleep that she has missed out on anyway, so it won't matter if she falls asleep earlier. Let her sleep on until the usual wake-up time of 10–10:15 a.m. If she is still sleeping at this time then wake her up.

If she has woken between 7 and 7:30 a.m. she should be able to make it through to around 8:40 a.m. before needing to nap. Put her down swaddled (if that is what she likes) in her Moses basket or cot with lights out and curtains closed in a quiet room. If she cries then pick her up and check for wind and resettle her with a cuddle or the pat-and-shhh technique discussed later on in this chapter.

Most babies love this nap and would happily sleep much longer than the time suggested. If she is still sleeping at 10 a.m. then it is important that you go in and wake her around 10:15 a.m. This will ensure she is tired enough to sleep well at the big lunchtime sleep and she is also ready for her next feed.

10:30/11 a.m. Breast- or bottle-feed

A nappy change and a quick wash from head to toe (known as top and tailing), plus an outfit change into 'day clothes' if desired can be done when she wakes up before the next feed.

This morning nap will need to be gradually reduced in length as it will begin to affect how well she sleeps during her lunchtime sleep. The start time will always remain the same, between 8:40 and 9 a.m., but as she gets older you can reduce the amount of time she is asleep for by waking her earlier. You should reduce by 10 minutes every time her lunchtime nap is affected for more than three days in a row. This should then encourage her to sleep better and more soundly again. Eventually this morning nap will drop altogether and your baby will be able to make it through from her 7–8 a.m. wake-up time to her lunchtime nap at 11:45 a.m.

Lunchtime nap

This is the most important nap of the day and will remain as a crucial part of your baby's routine for the next two years at least, long after other naps are no longer needed. This sleep should be established and continued in the room where she usually sleeps at night – in her Moses basket or cot – as much as possible, to allow her a quality sleep in the most relaxed environment. Your baby can sleep in the pushchair or car seat for this sleep occasionally if you have family commitments that take you away from the family home over the lunchtime period. However it is important to allow her to have this sleep in the cot or Moses basket as much as possible. In my experience a baby never sleeps for as long when out and about and napping in a pushchair or car seat. You also don't want her falling into the habit of only ever sleeping when 'on the move' in a car seat or pushchair. This will lead to bad sleep associations and cat-napping.

A baby who sleeps well at lunchtime is much happier for the rest of the afternoon, meaning your afternoon nap and evening routine is also more likely to run smoothly. She will sleep better and wake feeling refreshed and in a better mood if she has had a good sleep in a quiet environment.

It is also very important to encourage your baby to establish one long sleep at some point during the day, so that she learns how to self-settle as she moves through the various stages of sleep. This will make a big difference to how well she settles and sleeps at night-time.

Babies who get into the habit of cat-napping during the day tend to wake up once they come into a light sleep. This will be a habit that continues into the night hours, and she will continue to wake up several times a night, every time she comes into a light sleep, and rely on you to help her get back to sleep again. This will not happen if you establish a long regular daily lunchtime sleep. It should always be a minimum of two hours long, but can be up to two and three-quarters or even three hours for some babies. The start time of 11:40/45 will always remain the same in the early stages.

If you find that your baby begins waking halfway through the nap on a regular basis and seems genuinely hungry, then a small top-up feed can be given, particularly if she is going through a growth spurt. Try the resettling techniques discussed first, before resorting to feeding. Do the top-up in the same room that your baby is sleeping, though, and treat it like a night feed, by keeping quiet, avoiding too much eye contact and encouraging her to go back to sleep afterwards until she has had a minimum of two hours' sleep.

If she begins waking regularly halfway through her nap, isn't particularly hungry or rooting around, but seems wide-awake and not wanting to go back to sleep, then it is time to reduce the morning nap. Equally, if she takes a long time to settle when you put her to bed at 11:45 it could also be due to having slept for too long in the morning.

Wake her up 10 minutes earlier than you would usually. This should be enough to encourage her to start sleeping better during her lunchtime nap again. If she still continues to wake halfway through then try to take a little more time off, as long as she is still able to make it through to the start time of this nap without dozing off.

Other things to consider that may be the cause of her waking early are:

- Wind
- Soiled nappy
- Teething (see Chapter 7 for more details)

Some babies will wake naturally just after 2 p.m. Other babies who need that extra sleep on a daily basis will carry on sleeping.

2:30 p.m. Breast- or bottle-feed
Wake her by 2:30 p.m. if she is still sleeping so that you can keep your feeds on track. Even if she has had an unsettled sleep from waking due to one reason or another you will still need to wake her at 2:30 p.m. to enable the rest of your afternoon to run smoothly.

As she gets older and drops her other naps she may enjoy a longer sleep at this time. As long as you always have her awake by 3pm then her bedtime routine shouldn't be affected.

Teatime nap
How long your baby needs to sleep at this time will greatly depend on how long she slept at lunchtime. This nap does not have to be

a solid sleep or in the Moses basket or cot in the dark, although some babies and parents prefer it that way.

If your baby is happy to doze on and off for a few 10–15-minute naps between 3:30 and 5:30 p.m. that is absolutely fine. I wouldn't suggest that you let her sleep solidly for that entire time over the age of six weeks, unless she had a very poor lunchtime nap and needs to make up for the sleep she has missed out on.

If she slept very well at lunchtime and had to be woken at 2:30 p.m. then she may happily make it through to 4 p.m. before needing to nap again. I always suggest an outing at this time. By this point in the day most mothers are getting cabin fever if they have been stuck in all day. I always found that putting the baby in the pram or pushchair at this time was good for everyone, particularly if you have a toddler as well as a baby. I used to really look forward to my afternoon walk when all three of my children were small babies. The walk usually means that the baby is almost guaranteed to sleep at some point too, which will stop her being grumpy and overtired before the bath and bedtime routine begins. Try to ensure that she doesn't wake before 5 p.m. so that you are able to stick to the two-hour sleep rule between 5 p.m. and bedtime, which will prevent her becoming overtired.

As she gets older, more alert and interested in her surroundings, then a walk may not send her off to sleep at this time any more. She will be far more interested in looking around her. If she is of an age where you think she can manage to last without a teatime nap then it can be dropped. If she still shows signs of needing it then a car journey at the right time to run an errand or get some shopping will usually send her off to sleep; alternatively some babies just prefer to have this sleep in the cot until they are ready to drop it.

Babies who are a bit sleepier than others may not last until 4 p.m. You may find that she dozes off around 3:30 p.m. – particularly if breastfed, as she may fall asleep at the end of the feed. If this happens, then you can split her naps. Allow her half an hour if she dozes before 4 p.m., then rouse her and wake her up. It's important that you then encourage her to have another 15–30 minutes' sleep closer to 5 p.m. to prevent overtiredness. If she has had the earlier sleep then bring your 5 p.m. feed forward to 4:45 p.m. and she will doze off after that.

Wake her by 5:30 p.m.
4:45/5:00 p.m.: Feed, depending on sleeps discussed above

5:30/5:45 p.m.: Bath or top and tail and change into night clothes
A bath does tend to make a baby relaxed so where possible try to make this a regular part of your evening routine.

6:00/6:30 p.m.: Full breast or bottle-feed in a quiet calm environment

6:45/7:00 p.m.: In bed, settled and asleep

Bedtime sleep 6:45/7 p.m.–10/10:45 p.m.
This sleep should definitely be in the Moses basket or cot in a dark, quiet room. In my experience this is the part of the day that all babies fight the most, and is the hardest sleep to establish. It usually takes a period of weeks to get your baby sleeping reliably from 7–10 p.m. without her waking up at all.

Here are some tips to enable you to establish this sleep effectively and quickly:

- Ensure she has had a nap somewhere between 4 and 5 p.m. The time this happens and the length will be individual to your baby. You need to establish what works best for her, and this can also change from day to day, depending on how well she slept at lunchtime.
- Give her a bath before her last feed as this will help wind her down. A massage can also sometimes help.

- Put her to bed in her Moses basket or cot in a quiet dark room away from all TV noise and other children.
- If she wakes after a period of time asleep, wind is probably the problem in the first few weeks. Pick her up, wind her and try to resettle her back to sleep again.
- If she was particularly sleepy during her last feed, she may not have fed effectively and may wake due to hunger. If you think this is possible then offer her the breast again to resettle her if you are breastfeeding. If you are formula feeding, then she can be offered a bottle top-up any time up to 8 p.m. without it having a major impact on her next feed, although I would advise you doing the next feed closer to 11 p.m. if you do have to top-up. Offer the feed in her room rather than bringing

---

Tip

If you have been trying for a long period of time from 7 p.m. onwards to settle your baby back to sleep and, despite winding, topping up and checking her nappy, she still hasn't settled to sleep, it is most likely that your window of sleep has passed and she has become overtired. In this instance she will continue to be unsettled until she has her 10–11 p.m. feed. This feed usually encourages a baby to fall straight to sleep afterwards if they feed well. If you can manage to get her to doze at least in your arms before you give her the feed, then she will feed more effectively. If she is too exhausted by the time her last feed is offered then the risk is that she will only take a minimal amount and then fall straight to sleep. If this happens, then the result will be that she will be so hungry in the night she will probably end up demanding an extra feed. It is worth persevering in trying to get her to drink a reasonable amount of milk and take a good feed between 10 and 11 p.m. to prevent extra night waking. Nappy changes, tickling and undressing should all help keep her awake enough to feed effectively.

her into the living room in a potentially noisy stimulating environment. This will wake her up more and make it much harder to settle her back to sleep immediately afterwards. After feeding, wind her as normal and resettle her back to sleep in her Moses basket or cot.

Patience and Perseverance

You may find that in the first few weeks of establishing this sleep that you and your partner are regularly going to and fro to settle your baby. Remember the two Ps: patience and perseverance. If you are consistent, things will improve and soon you will have time to enjoy a relaxing evening again, with a baby happily sleeping and settled upstairs in her cot. If you do bring her out of the nursery and downstairs on a regular basis, then she will get used to that and be less likely to want to go back to sleep.

All of the information in this book is meant as a guide only and to give you an idea of what is a normal and healthy amount of sleep for a baby at various ages. I have heard a few people recommend to new mums to keep their baby awake as much as possible during the day, and then she will sleep better at night. This is very far from the truth. A very young baby who is forced to stay awake for long periods of time will be grumpy and irritable and be more unsettled during the night as a result. With a small baby, sleep promotes sleep if structured in the correct way. A baby will find it a lot easier to doze off and sleep well if she is given the correct calm environment, and is not too fractious or overtired to settle.

I'm sure you are aware yourself of those times when you are so exhausted due to family or work commitments, you look forward to going to bed and assume you will go straight to sleep because you are so tired. Instead you find yourself lying there watching the clock, hour after hour, willing yourself to fall asleep but not able to. The more tired and frustrated you feel, the harder it is to relax enough to fall asleep. Babies are exactly the same, and the more overtired they get, the harder they, and you, will find it is to get them to go to sleep and settle down into a relaxed sleep, rather than a fitful one.

During the first eight to ten weeks it is very important that you stick to the two-hour rule where your baby's sleep is concerned. If she is down and asleep within two hours of the last time she woke, then she should never get to the overtired stage. There will, of course, be times when wind, unexpected nappy changes or last-minute top-up feeds may push you past this two-hour limit. Occasionally you may get away with it and she may settle off to sleep. However, more often than not you will enter a cycle of crying and being unsettled, where she becomes more and more overtired the longer she stays awake. Unfortunately, you just have to ride out these moments until she is finally so exhausted that she goes to sleep.

Her ability to stay awake for longer periods of time will increase as she gets older. By the age of eight to ten weeks a baby can usually cope with the two-hour rule, stretching to two and a half or even three hours between naps before they reach the overtired meltdown. You will need to gauge this with your individual baby.

The part of the day this usually happens at is the afternoon, between her lunchtime nap and teatime nap. You may notice, for example, if she woke at 2 p.m. and then dozed off again around 4:30/5 p.m. she was perfectly happy for that period of time.

As her age increases over the next few months she will eventually drop her teatime nap and not need it any more. At this point you will find she probably falls asleep regularly on her 6–7 p.m. milk feed. It varies as to the age a baby is ready to drop this nap but it is somewhere between 6 and 12 months. It will be obvious that she doesn't need it any more by the fact that she doesn't go to sleep on a walk or car journey, or just chats when she is put in her cot at that time.

It varies from baby to baby, and even between siblings or twins, when they are ready to increase the time between naps or drop them altogether.

The naptimes that I have given you are a guide. So many parents are unsure how much sleep a baby should have on a daily basis or even when to time the sleeps. The structures of sleeps that I have suggested give you something to try. It is down to you to fine-tune the times to fit in with your family and life commitments. If you have school runs for example with older siblings then the times that I have suggested may not work for you entirely. In the early days and weeks a baby usually always falls asleep while on the move in the pushchair or a car journey.

The best solution in these instances is to split their naptime if you have a school or nursery run which means your baby is likely to fall asleep on the journey but the sleep would be too early for the suggested guide sleep times.

Below I have given an example of how to adapt your baby's sleep times when you need to incorporate a school or nursery run with older children.

1: School run in the car: **8:15–9:15 a.m.**
2: Nursery run at **12–12:30 p.m.** in the pushchair or car
3: School run at **3–3:45 p.m.** in the pushchair or car

1: Your baby will almost certainly sleep for the entire ride or car journey when she is very small. I would suggest you wake her when you arrive home at 9:15 a.m. You can top and tail her or change her nappy to rouse her. If she wants to, or you can encourage her, to doze again around 10 a.m. for 10–15 minutes, this would be ideal. She should then be able to last until her next naptime at around 11:45 a.m. If she doesn't have the extra doze around 10 a.m. then she will probably end up dozing off during or immediately after her 10:30 a.m. feed. Allow her to sleep for 15–30 minutes and then try rousing her, again with a nappy change or by removing some of her clothes. Encourage her to finish the remainder of her feed if she fell asleep partway through and then wind her back down ready for her full lunchtime nap around 12 p.m. Depending on how long she dozed back off for and at what time, you may need to adapt the time at which she is ready to go back off to sleep at lunchtime. As long as you ensure that you stick to the two-hour rule where her sleep is concerned so that she doesn't become overtired, she should happily settle back to sleep for her long lunchtime nap.

2: Your baby may fall asleep again on this second car or pushchair journey. As this is her long lunchtime naptime anyway it would be ideal if she stayed asleep once you returned home. If she is in the pushchair then I would suggest you leave her in a quiet dark room somewhere to continue sleeping until the suggested wake-up time of 2–2:30 p.m. If she fell asleep in the car seat then you can attempt to transfer her to the Moses basket or cot on your return home, again in a quiet, dark room, to continue sleeping.

3: Depending on how well she slept over lunchtime she may or may not fall asleep at this time. If she does, then wake her as soon as you can. Again, you can rouse her by undressing her and doing a nappy change, and then try to keep her awake for a little while. She should then need another short nap around 5 p.m. If she is under eight weeks and still having the 5 p.m. top-up feed then you could try offering her the top-up at 4:45 p.m. This will then make her sleepy and encourage her to doze off. Wake her by 5:30 p.m. at the latest to begin your bath, milk and bedtime routine to aim for a 7 p.m. bedtime.

Even if you have had a rough day of your baby being unsettled and not sleeping a great deal, the most important sleep to try to get right is the teatime nap between 4 and 5:30 p.m. If you can encourage her to nap somewhere between these times then she will be much easier to get settled down for the evening and sleep well between 7 and 10 p.m. A walk or a car journey are usually one of the two guaranteed methods to ensure your baby settles at this time, if you know you really need to get her to have a good nap.

I have read so many books and heard various professionals when advising on childcare issues say, 'never do this, never do that.'

When you are a parent there is hardly ever a situation where you will be able to say that you will never do something and stick to it forever. There will come a time when every parent ends up breaking their own parenting rules for a bit of peace and quiet or because it is what your baby needs at that particular moment in time and nothing else is likely to work.

I always tell the parents that I work with to trust their instincts for what will work on the odd occasions, without creating bad habits by continuing to do something repeatedly. Doing something as a one-off is fine. It is if you repeat it three or more times that it can develop into a habit that your baby will learn to expect every time.

If your baby is teething or unwell then your usual parenting rules will have to be relaxed. Your baby will need more cuddles and attention at times like this. Try to stick to your usual daily routine as much as possible, but be prepared to adapt. Once your baby is on the mend and feeling herself again, then you can all aim to get things back to normal again.

Conditions affecting sleep

Flat head syndrome

The technical name for this condition is **plagiocephaly** but it is more commonly known as flat head syndrome. The most common form is positional plagiocephaly, which occurs when a baby's head develops a flat spot due to continued pressure on that area. Because babies spend so much time lying on their back when asleep for example, they may develop a flat spot where their head presses against the mattress. Experts have noticed a five-fold increase in misshapen heads since the advice to sleep babies on their backs came into force. Another type of plagiocephaly is craniosynostosis, which is a birth defect in which the skull bones join too early (see fontanelle section in Chapter 3 on page 57). Babies born with this will need surgery to allow their brain to grow properly.

More rarely babies can develop positional plagiocephaly when movement in the uterus is restricted for some reason, e.g., the mother is carrying more than one baby or a breech baby becomes wedged under the mother's ribs.

Many naturally delivered babies have a misshapen head for the first few weeks, particularly if you had an assisted delivery, e.g., forceps or ventouse. This usually corrects itself by the age of six weeks, but if you still feel it is misshapen after this age, or you have only just noticed a flat spot, then it is more likely to be due to your baby's sleeping position.

If you do notice a flat spot from an early age, it will be helpful to take a photo regularly to observe any changes.

It is well worth mentioning your worries to your GP sooner rather than later. It is much easier to correct the condition while your baby is still young and the skull is soft and pliable. This becomes less so the older your baby gets, as her skull bones begin to fuse together in her two fontanelles.

In many cases a doctor may advise that you wait until your baby is over the age of six months, because any soft spot may round out on its own by then as your baby begins to sit up and crawl. If you have ensured that you have regularly changed your baby's sleeping/sitting/feeding position and the flat spot hasn't improved, then your doctor is likely to recommend that your baby is fitted with a custom fitted helmet to correct the shape of her head. This has to be worn for 23 hours a day and the treatment generally lasts two to six months, depending on the age it starts and the severity of the flat spot.

The idea of your baby wearing something around or on her head on an almost permanent basis sounds terrifying to any parent. However, the helmets are very lightweight and, when fitted on a young baby, they get used to them very quickly and don't have any sleep issues related to the helmet.

Out of all the babies I have worked with, just one has had to be fitted with one of these helmets. His head circumference was noted by the health visitor and doctors as being larger than an average baby's head from when he was first born. It was then regularly monitored and never settled down. Both his mother and I ensured he had regular positional changes during his daytime play and at night, but he had to be fitted with his helmet at the age of six months. He adapted amazingly well to it within the first 24 hours, and had to wear it for the recommended 23 hours per day for just over nine months. It was removed for an hour at bath time every day and then put back on in time for bed. Nine months after having it fitted his head shape had normalised.

Wind

The biggest cause that tends to make a baby unsettled at night and less likely to go to sleep is wind. Even if she hasn't had any kind of wind issues during the day that does not mean you can rule it out as a reason for a difficult night. Wind is more likely to cause a problem and affect how settled a baby is at night because they have to lie down for a much longer period of time. Lying her on her side, rather than her back, to sleep will help make her feel more comfortable and help her settle back to sleep immediately after a feed. You can also place a towel or blanket under the top end of her mattress where her head lies, to elevate her sleeping position. Another option, if you would prefer not to do that, is to put books under the two feet of her Moses basket or cot, at the head end to elevate her sleeping position. This is the best position for her to lie in so that wind doesn't trouble her so much and cause her to keep waking up. It is also a good position for babies suffering from reflux or colic (see page 114 and 108).

You may hear her grunting and making noises as she sleeps. This is usually a sign that she has wind if she is generally a quiet or silent sleeper. If you begin to hear her grunting and squeaking in her sleep and it starts to get louder and more frequent, rather than just a continual noise at the same level, then it is a good idea to pick her up and check for a burp by placing her over your shoulder to wind. If she does have wind then she is likely to burp within a minute or two of you patting her back. As she is still asleep or half asleep when you do this she should be happy to go straight back down again and continue sleeping without the squeaks and grunts. If you ignore this consistent noise that begins to get louder, it is likely that she will wake herself up and cry as she needs you to pick her up and wind her, because it has become too uncomfortable to sleep through. It will then be more difficult to resettle her, particularly if it is not her usual feed time, because she has woken up fully.

Equally, if you ignore her grunting, the danger is that she will vomit. If a burp is left 'festering away' and you ignore the signs that your baby has wind, then it tends to make its way out somehow. Air bubbles become trapped under any extra milk she had after they were formed and they then push the milk upwards and cause her to be sick. She will then panic, which is a perfectly normal reaction, and need you to pick her up, mop up the vomit and calm her down by reassuring her with your voice. This whole scenario will wake your baby fully and make it difficult to settle her again. That is why it is a good idea to pick her up to check for wind if she does seem to be increasing her grunting noises or wriggling around a lot.

If it is just a continual grunt or squeak and she is moving around regularly, then it may just be her way of sleeping and getting herself comfortable. Just as adults move around in the bed and roll over in our sleep, many babies are also very wriggly too. Some babies also grunt anyway and they are fairly noisy sleepers. It doesn't always mean they have wind, and will sometimes snore, grunt and squeak every time they are asleep without you ever needing to worry that wind is causing it. As long as it is a consistent noise that is normal for your baby, then don't worry. You are looking for something out of the ordinary.

Winding after the 10:30 p.m. feed

After the 10:30 p.m. feed always spend at least 20 minutes with your baby over your shoulder to wind her. This helps the milk to settle down and gives time for as much wind as possible to come up before you put her down and try to get the longest stretch of sleep out of her. Babies usually fall asleep immediately after this feed anyway, but by just sitting somewhere quietly with them over your shoulder, you can pat their back every few minutes or so, to ensure you get all of the wind. It is a good idea to repeat this 20-minute winding process after the night feed too and after any feed where you are planning on putting her straight to sleep afterwards, although this 10:30 p.m. feed winding process will be the most essential.

It is very tempting to put a baby down to sleep very quickly after the late or night feed as you will be feeling very tired yourself at this time. However, by putting your baby down too quickly while she still has some wind, you may end up getting less sleep as she is more likely to be unsettled. She may shuffle around in her sleep, be grunting and noisy and then eventually cry as the wind is too uncomfortable to sleep with any more. This means that you could end up jumping in and out of bed like a yo-yo, as you pick her up three or four times, trying to get the last bits of wind that were missed.

- The method I always use at the 10:30 p.m. feed is to sit and wind after the feed for around 20 minutes. Put the baby over your shoulder and pat her back every few minutes to check for wind. Rub her back every now and then in between.
- At the end of the 20 minutes or so, get her swaddled and put her down in her Moses basket or cot.
- If she begins wriggling and grunting immediately then pick her up and put her over your shoulder again and pat her back to check for wind. Put her back down again once she is calm.

- If she is still sleeping and not wriggly at the point of you putting her down then I usually go and get my pyjamas on, go to the bathroom and brush my teeth. This extra five minutes of lying down gives her body a chance to allow any wind that is almost ready to come up, to get where it needs to be.

- Once I am ready for bed I then go back in to the baby. At this point, even if she isn't wriggling, squeaking or grunting, and is sleeping soundly I **always** pick her up one last time and put her over my shoulder to pat her back. Half the time you will find that they end up doing another burp. It is always worth checking that last time before you settle down for the night. Even if your baby is asleep as you pick her up, you will not wake her, and ensuring that you have done your utmost to get all of the wind out will hopefully mean she, and you, will get a better stretch of sleep!

Crying and what causes it

All babies cry for a reason. Your job as a parent is to work out what the cause is and fix the problem, so that your baby feels happier and the crying stops. There are many different things that can cause your baby to cry:

- Hunger
- A wet or soiled nappy
- Being tired or overtired
- Overstimulation
- Being bored
- Feeling uncomfortable
- Tummy pain or constipation
- Wind
- Teething

- General pain
- Illnesses or just feeling unwell

Although any of the above can cause a baby to cry, the four main causes of crying in a newborn or very young baby are: hunger, a wet or soiled nappy, wind or being overtired.

These four possible causes need to be at the top of your radar when your baby cries. So when she starts to cry, think of these things:

1: Does she have a wet or soiled nappy?
2: Does she have wind? Put her over your shoulder and pat to check for any immediate wind that may come up as a burp.
3: Is she still hungry? Does she need a top-up feed if she didn't feed particularly well, or is she just looking to suck for comfort – in which case she can be offered the dummy.
4: Has she been awake too long and got herself overtired? Remember to stick to the two-hour rule in a baby under eight weeks.

If you are sure that none of the main things suggested are causing the crying then it is worth investigating the other causes of crying on the list.

Up to the age of around five to six weeks babies are not manipulative. A newborn baby will cry for a reason. As her parent, you need to respond to that cry as quickly and as effectively as you can, and try to eliminate the problem. As soon as you manage to do this, the crying will stop. Sounds simple right? If you have a daily structure it makes it easier to identify the cause of any crying.

The babies that I work with cry very little, and that is because they simply don't need to. Their every need is met on a daily basis in terms of feeding and sleeping, which makes it easier to work out the cause of any crying.

A baby who is fed on demand and just left to doze as and when will be much harder to entertain and keep happy, than a baby who has a daily routine.

If you are demand feeding on the breast every one to two hours then your baby will definitely feel hungry a lot of the day in spite of the regular feeds. This is due to her not obtaining enough of the fatty hind milk at each feed. It is comparable to you snacking on salad and fruit all day as opposed to being offered a few hearty filling meals. Understandably, that is likely to make her fairly cranky and irritable on a daily basis and continue to need to feed frequently to satisfy her hunger.

Equally if she is cat-napping all day for 30–60 minutes at a time, she will very quickly end up overtired. It is so important to encourage good sleeping habits from a very young age. A quality amount and length of sleep is good for us all, and your baby will be in a much better mood from day to day if her feeds and sleep are structured as much as possible.

If you ensure that your baby's sleep and feeding needs are met regularly and effectively then you can usually eliminate those two reasons for her crying.

Babies do tend to have cries that sound slightly different to the trained ear, which mean different things. The main carer, usually the mother, can, with time, learn to distinguish between her baby's cries and what each one means.

This is only usually possible when your baby has a daily structure and feeds and sleeps are at similar times each day. If she doesn't have a routine then she will probably cry a fair amount on a daily basis anyway, as she will be hungry and tired a lot of the time.

If you are hearing your baby cry frequently on a daily basis then it will be a lot more difficult to learn to understand the differences between the cries and their meanings. One cry will blend into the next, and you really won't be concentrating on what the cry means if it just goes on and on.

The biggest cause of crying in a baby with no routine is usually overtiredness. Structuring sleep times will help every other aspect of her day and make her a much happier baby. The whole world seems a much brighter place when you are not facing a constant battle with overtiredness – this is true for all of us and our little ones from the start. I'm sure as a new parent you can also relate to this. If you sleep well or get a few hours of sleep in a row, it seems so much easier to cope. Routine is helpful for the following reasons:

- Your baby will feed better if she isn't so tired, as she will be more alert and feel refreshed from her regular daily naps.
- If she is feeding well and in bigger quantities rather than snack feeding at frequent intervals then she is less likely to suffer from as much wind or colic.
- She is also less likely to get either bored or overstimulated if she is getting a regular amount of sleep.

It is a win-win situation, and promoting good sleeping habits from a young age will mean your baby grows into a toddler and older child who continues to settle and sleep well for as long as you encourage it. Babies and children learn what they are taught where sleep is concerned. Remember that all babies have the potential to be 'good sleepers'. With lots of patience and perseverance yours can be one of them.

Crying caused by pain

A baby's pain cry is like no other you will hear. It is a piercing cry compared to their other cries and is even more heart-wrenching than their normal hungry or bored cry.

The first time most parents experience this new cry is when teething begins, so any time from around eight to ten weeks. It is always such a shock the first time you hear this new cry, and teething is sometimes forgotten as a potential cause as the cry can come so unexpectedly at a fairly young age. A baby with teething pain or experiencing any other type of pain will cry inconsolably and will not be soothed no matter what a parent does. No amount of cuddling will relieve the problem – it may comfort your baby and the cries subside every now and then, but they will resume crying again until the pain is taken away.

Pain relief in the form of infant paracetamol like Calpol or Nurofen for Children will relieve the pain, but should only be given if your baby is old enough, usually around the age of 12 weeks, and you are sure that teething pain is the cause. If you are not sure and worried then take your baby to your doctor and get her checked over. More information on teething signs and symptoms can be found in Chapter 7, page 267.

Once you eliminate and solve the cause of a baby's crying she should be much easier to settle. Up to the age of five to six weeks most babies need help to settle to sleep. There are only a very small percentage of babies under this age who are able to settle themselves from being put down wide-awake to drifting off to sleep. By all means try it with your baby at the naptimes suggested, but don't be surprised if she needs a bit of comfort and help from you.

If she cries it is very important that you respond to her. I don't advise any of the parents I work with to try the 'cry-it-out' method with any baby under the age of five to six weeks as it is unlikely to work. You may find on the odd occasion your baby will settle off to sleep after a few minutes of crying if you weren't able to get to her straight away – maybe if you were washing up or in the shower for example. On these occasions it is fine that she has had a little cry and managed to settle herself if you were busy, but, as a rule, it is important to go to her as soon as possible. In the long term it will make her a more independent, confident baby, secure in the knowledge that when she is really upset then someone will come to her.

The aim is to get your baby from wide-awake to a drowsy state before attempting to put her down for a nap. She will then learn to drop off into a deep sleep on her own with time, rather than relying on you to always help her get there.

There are various ways to achieve this:

- Breast- or bottle-feeding generally makes a very young baby sleepy towards the end of a feed when her tummy is feeling full and she isn't holding on to any excess wind. This is particularly useful after the 6 p.m., 10.30 p.m. and night feed, as the aim is for her to go straight to sleep afterwards anyway. It is important not to fall into the trap of always 'feeding her to sleep', though, as this will create a sleep association that will need to be changed later on. At the evening and night feeds it is inevitable that she will be much more sleepy anyway and likely to doze by the end of the feed. However, try to keep her more alert during the day feeds, and pause the feed midway to wake her slightly if she seems to be sleeping on the bottle or at the breast.

- Offering your baby a dummy can help to get her from wide-awake to a drowsy state. It is important that you take the dummy away before she drops into a deep sleep with it in her mouth, still sucking it. This will prevent her becoming dependent on it, and then needing to rely on it as a sleep prop to get herself to sleep, or to resettle herself every time she comes into a light sleep. The aim is that, whatever method you use to get her drowsy, as she gets older she then learns to do the last part of settling herself into a deep sleep on her own. Eventually she will be able to settle herself off to sleep from being wide-awake and put down in her cot.

- Swaddle her and then cuddle her in your arms using the pat-and-shhh technique below. At times you may need to also use the dummy to begin with if she is wide-awake. You can attempt to remove the dummy once she is looking sleepy and continue with the 'pat-and-shhh' technique before placing her in her Moses basket or cot.

The 'pat-and-shhh' technique

Swaddle your baby, or wrap her however she prefers in the basket or cot. If she is lying on her right side, gently pat her bottom in a heartbeat rhythm: pat pat, pat pat, pat pat, pat pat. As you do this make a shhh, shhh, sound with your mouth. If she is lying on her back, you can either pat her tummy gently or pat the side of the top of her leg. These two things combined remind your baby of being in the womb, where she was listening to your heart beating and your blood whooshing around. If she is unsettled and rooting around as you do this, then you can try putting the dummy in her mouth as you continue to pat and shhh.

Once her body movements calm down and she seems more relaxed, then you can remove the dummy, but continue with the patting and shushing. It is important that you only take away one comfort at a time. If you were to stop everything all at once then she would definitely notice and probably begin to wake herself fully again.

Allowing your baby to experience these comforts will not make her develop bad sleep association habits at this young age. It will actually aid her ability to settle herself much easier once she is over the age of six weeks, because she will feel secure that you respond to her cries.

- If she begins fussing again once you remove the dummy, and becomes more unsettled with just the patting and shushing, then give her the dummy back again and continue for another five minutes.
- After five minutes try removing the dummy again. Once it is successfully removed then continue with the patting and shushing. Pause the shhing every now and then, and if she remains settled then stop saying it altogether, but continue the heartbeat rhythm pat.
- Once you are left with only the patting then you can begin to slow it down. Continue with the heartbeat rhythm but miss a beat every now and then. Keep on doing this until you manage to stop it altogether. If she becomes unsettled again then add the shhh noise back in, if needed, and then take away when appropriate.
- Leave your hand resting on her bottom for a minute or two after you have stopped patting and then gradually remove the pressure, lifting your hand away as she sleeps.

- If she begins to wriggle again then try just adding in the shhh shhh noise rather than patting her again.
- If it all goes wrong then you may have to begin all over again, or even pick her up for a cuddle before putting her back in the basket again. If she is very wriggly it can sometimes indicate excess wind, which will definitely prevent her from settling to sleep. Pick her up and put her over your shoulder and pat her back to wind her. Then you can attempt to resettle her back in her basket or cot.

The above may sound slightly complicated to begin with, but it really isn't, and, with instinct and practice, it is a very simple and effective method to use. There will of course be times that it takes a few attempts to get your baby to settle. Equally other times you may find she settles as soon as you put her down without any need to pat or shhh.

It is always worth encouraging the minimum of help from you in settling her, but if she does cry then she needs to be sure that you will respond to that. In reassuring and comforting her with cuddles and attention when she needs it during the first few weeks of her life, she will respond much better when you get to the stage after six weeks of encouraging her to learn to settle herself more of the time.

CASE STUDY: The pat-and-shhh technique in action

I had a call from a mother called Victoria when her baby was four weeks old. Max was her second child and she called me because he was crying a lot during the day and night-time when it was time to go to sleep. Having had a child previously who had slipped into bad habits from an early age, Victoria didn't want the same to happen with Max. She thought that if she taught him to self-soothe from newborn, he would end up learning much quicker, sleep better, and not learn the wrong sleep associations. He happily fed well from the bottle and didn't seem to suffer from excess or trapped wind. However, at four weeks Max was a very unhappy baby when it came to being put down or going to sleep. Victoria would put him down from awake and leave him to cry to settle himself. Very occasionally he would settle himself but more often than not he would get himself so wound up that she would have to go to him to try to calm him down. By that stage he was usually so irate at being left to cry and thoroughly overtired that he refused to settle to sleep for hours anyway. Once she finally managed to get him to settle he would wake frequently, crying.

Victoria was passed my name by a friend and called me for some advice. As soon as she told me the age of Max and that she had been leaving him to self-soothe as much as possible from birth I realised that was the problem.

It is very important that you don't try to encourage your baby to settle herself to sleep during the early days and weeks by using the cry-it-out method. With 99 per cent of babies it will not work if they are under the age of four weeks. The only result will be that she becomes more and more irate, and gets very upset that no one is responding to her. There are a minority of babies who are able to settle themselves and have a very short crying bout of around one to two minutes before going off to sleep. You may notice your baby does manage to do this every now and then if you haven't quite managed to get to her as soon as she starts crying, as you are busy with something else or older siblings.

If you continue the cry-it-out method over time then it sends your baby the message that her crying will be ignored whenever she is put down to sleep. This turns her into a very fractious, clingy baby who wants to make the most of being held frequently, as she will think that every time she is put down that no one will respond to her. She will therefore crave even more attention. This is what had happened with Max.

I immediately told her that she had to go back to basics with Max and treat him like a newborn in terms of getting him off to sleep. He should be held frequently and whenever it was time to go to sleep she should swaddle him and then cuddle him until he was very dozy. She should then use the pat-and-shhh technique to help him drift off to sleep. If he cried while settling she should respond to it as quickly as possible by picking him up to soothe and reassure him. We booked in a few weeks *of nights for me to help out as Victoria was exhausted from the first few weeks after birth.*

Within a few days Max was a much happier baby, and responded well to the extra attention. Victoria found it much easier to settle him to sleep and he was sleeping for much longer stretches, particularly at night, which had previously been their worst time.

After a couple of weeks he was following the feeding and sleep routine very well so we began to try to put him down a little less drowsy to settle him to sleep. As he was now in such a good routine Victoria had become very good at understanding the difference between his hungry and tired cries. He again responded very well, and over the next couple of weeks got even better at settling himself so that he was then able to settle himself from wide-awake. As he was now eight weeks and had regained his confidence in knowing that someone would come to him if needed, then it was okay to let him try to self-soothe for a short period of time.

I told Victoria that it was still very important she respond to him if he didn't seem to be settling and his crying increased rather than decreased. This could mean he had wind or just needed an extra cuddle or she could use the pat-and-shhh technique to reassure him. Over the next two weeks he also dropped his night feed by gradually sleeping for longer periods at night too.

Co-sleeping

During the first few days, nights and weeks you may find that co-sleeping during certain points of the night will help your baby to feel more settled. It is always a good plan to begin the evening and night with her sleeping in her Moses basket or cot. If she becomes unsettled during the night and wakes earlier than her usual feed time, but refuses to settle back in the basket after a cuddle, then a cuddle in the bed next to you, where she can feel the warmth and comfort of your body and smell, will most definitely help soothe her back to sleep.

Co-sleeping, even if only for short bursts of time, is a totally personal choice. No doubt you will be plagued with the worry that you may accidentally smother your baby. Statistically the chances of this are very rare. In the UK, around 300 babies die of cot death per year. Of these less than 1 per cent die of suffocation in their parents' bed and these deaths can be avoided, if parents:

- Don't smoke
- Avoid alcohol and any medications that cause drowsiness
- Don't fall asleep on the sofa with the baby (squashier than a bed so more likely to suffocate)
- Aren't extremely tired and ensure the baby doesn't get trapped under the quilt

Although most new parents would describe themselves as 'extremely tired', you only need to worry if you feel too tired to leave the house – if this is the case then you should avoid sleeping with your baby.

In my experience as a parent, and in talking to other mothers, you never properly sleep if your baby is next to you anyway. You just tend to doze and every little sound or movement they make is heard or felt, and you instinctively wake fully to check on them. Provided you take the above precautions then sleeping with your baby when needed appears safe.

The biggest question you need to ask yourself regarding co-sleeping is how would you feel if your baby were to die from cot death while in your bed? Would you be plagued with regret and guilt, despite the fact that your baby's death was highly unlikely to have been caused by bed-sharing? Although NHS midwives and health visitors will happily advise on safe co-sleeping, society at large is still wary of bed-sharing with babies. That in itself makes the decision about whether to take your baby into your bed even more complicated, and a totally personal choice.

CASE STUDY: My experience with co-sleeping

I didn't co-sleep with my babies all the time, only when I felt it was necessary, and they needed some extra comfort. This would usually be at a time when they had woken slightly earlier than their feed time and I wanted to stall them a little bit longer before I fed them. I would always try picking them up and winding them over my shoulder first. If they didn't resettle there with a cuddle and stay calm when I attempted to put them back in their bed, then I usually found a cuddle in bed next to me with the dummy would help to resettle them and keep them dozing until the feed time. As they were continuing to doze in the lead up to their feed this prevented them becoming overtired and more difficult to settle once I eventually did do the feed.

In my experience, all babies are generally quite unsettled between 5 and 7 a.m. in the morning, after a night feed. They come into more of a light sleep at that time, and the night feed also tends to give them extra wind, which can bother them for the remaining night period.

If your baby is always particularly windy anyway, then she may only settle lying on your chest or propped upright on a V-pillow after the night feed, as it will be more comfortable than lying flat in her Moses basket or cot. The introduction of Infacol or another form of infant colic relief can help your baby to feel more comfortable as the wind bubbles are broken down in her tummy more readily. This will make her easier to settle at night-time, even if she doesn't seem to be affected by wind during the daytime. The process of having to lie down for a long period of time at night means wind is more likely to affect your baby at this time. During the day, air bubbles tend to release themselves without too much effort because babies are more active.

In my experience co-sleeping is only needed on certain occasions until you drop the night feed. Once that feed is no longer required, babies tend to sleep much better, as the extra wind from the night feed is no longer an issue.

Initially your baby may stir, wake slightly and need to be resettled between 5 and 7 a.m. but you will find that she won't be looking for food or be desperately hungry before 7 a.m. A quick cuddle or use of the pat-and-shhh technique will usually be enough to resettle her. If needed, you can bring her into the bed for a cuddle to help her doze off next to you until 7/7:30 a.m.

Over the following two weeks after a night feed has been dropped, you should find that your baby sleeps more soundly, and will gradually start going through to 7 a.m. without waking at all. This is the best time to phase co-sleeping out completely to prevent your baby relying on it as she gets older. If at points over the next few weeks or months, she begins to wake early or in the night, it is not a good idea to bring her into your bed any more. If you do, she will very quickly get used to the routine of waking more frequently and expect to come into bed with you. An older baby or child is not usually a good sleep partner. Even if they sleep well, it is unlikely that you will, with them moving around and frequently jabbing little arms and legs in your face! If she does wake when ill or teething, it is a good idea to have a chair in her nursery. You can sit with her in there for a cuddle if she is unsettled and then put her in her cot to go back to sleep in her own sleep environment. If you always stick to this basic rule on a regular basis as she gets older, then she won't develop any bad sleep association where she expects to come into your bed each time she wakes.

Once the night feed has been dropped this is also the perfect time to phase out and stop using the dummy. If you have only been using the dummy as a stalling tactic for feeds and to get her drowsy as suggested, then she shouldn't be attached to it and no longer using it will not be a problem. As long as you stop use of a dummy by 12 weeks then your baby will not become attached to it and begin to rely on it. If you do keep using the dummy once your baby is over 12 weeks old then with each passing week your baby will become more and more attached to it and begin to rely on it as a sleep prop. She will eventually get to the stage where she begins to wake frequently at night and need to use it to get herself back to sleep every time she comes into a light sleep. If she is too young to move around the cot herself, then this will mean traipsing back and forward to her bedroom to keep putting the dummy back into her mouth again. Not a great habit to get into.

Sleep associations

It is a good idea to encourage certain sleep props or associations, as they will give your baby a cue that it is time to go to sleep. It also means that if she wakes early from a nap or in the middle of the night, then you can use the sleep prop, as described below, to encourage her to go back to sleep.

Muslin squares or comfort toys

There are various different tag blankets and teddies that are advertised for parents to give to their babies as a sleep comforter. Some of them are very cute and tempting to buy. The main problem with using a teddy or tag toy as a sleep comforter is the risk of losing it once your child is attached to it and relying on it as a form of getting herself to sleep. If you do choose to encourage your baby to become attached to this type of item, then it is very important that you buy two of them exactly the same. At least then, you will always have one in reserve if the main one get lost.

The other problem with having a teddy or tag toy as a comforter is the difficulty with washing it. Unless you are very organised and wash each one frequently, your baby will very easily be able to tell the difference between her regular, most used comforter and the one she uses less frequently. She will definitely be less inclined to accept the 'reserve comforter' if it is not given to her on a regular basis. Equally, teddies in particular can quickly become very smelly, especially if your baby is sick on it at some point, which is an almost certainty. The smell of vomit is impossible to get rid of on a cuddly toy, no matter how many times you wash it. Your baby won't mind, of course, but you and everyone else who touches it will find the smell revolting!

In my opinion, muslin squares make perfect comforters. They are made of thin, breathable, washable material and can be purchased in supermarkets, as well as baby department stores. They are also big enough to make it less likely that she will lose it while in her cot in the dark, although you can put more than one in with her to ensure she can find one easily. Muslin squares are a very practical item to use during feeding and winding, so your baby can get used to them from the day she is born.

If you are only half-swaddling her for sleep and naptimes, then you can give her a muslin to hold between her hands each time you put her down to sleep. Young babies love to grab and hold anything that is put into their hand, so she will feel really comforted holding on to the muslin as she sleeps. She will also be less likely to wake herself fully with the startle reflex if she has something to grip on to for comfort, as she startles.

It is a good idea to change the muslin on a daily basis and give her a fresh one. This will stop her getting used to exactly the same one all the time. They will all smell the same anyway, with them being washed using the same products.

Muslin squares are made from a breathable cotton material, so it is okay if she wants to keep it close to her face for comfort. Many babies enjoy doing this to get a better smell of the reassuring scent that they are used to. You can tuck half of the muslin down under the mattress if you are particularly worried about her putting it too close to her face when she is very young. As she gets older, she will be able to roll away or move her head if she doesn't like to have it too close to her face.

Encouraging her to become attached to a muslin for sleep times will also be a comfort to her when she is away from you or the family home, and being cared for by relatives or family friends. The muslin will smell familiar to her, and reassure her if she is feeling anxious or upset.

Cot mobile

The basic tune or music that a cot mobile provides can be used as a very effective cue to let your baby know it is time to go to sleep. You don't need an elaborate mobile with a full-on light show, especially as this is more likely to stimulate your baby to stay awake. A cot mobile can be used as a daily sleep association once you start to put your baby down more awake on a regular basis, which usually happens around the age of five to six weeks. Up to this age, you can get her used to the familiar tune of it by placing her under it to watch, as you run her bath for example. You can also use the cot mobile when you put her down for a nap, but it's more likely that under the age of five weeks she will usually be pretty sleepy by the time you put her in her Moses basket or cot. Winding the cot mobile up at that point may wake her up if she is already dozing. Use it when you think the time is right.

The process that I have always used with my three children is first to swaddle them or place them in their sleeping bag in the cot. I then close the curtains and turn the lights out and wind the mobile up as I leave the room. If you stick to this exact same routine every time you put your baby down for a nap, whether it is for a daytime or night-time sleep, she will very quickly learn to associate the mobile music as her cue to go to sleep. It will also comfort her to always have the same familiar routine as she is put to bed. This will mean she will settle to sleep much easier from being wide-awake than if you changed things every time you put her down.

If she does wake in the night after she has dropped her night feed, then after checking on her to see what could be causing the problem – wind, nappy or teething, for example – you can then wind the mobile up as you usually would before you go out of the room. This will act as a sign to her that it is still night-time and you want her to go back to sleep. The mobile can also be used in the case of a baby who wakes too early in the morning. Again, I would firstly suggest you go in and do your usual checks: nappy, wind, sleeping position. I would then give her any comforter she has, like a muslin or teddy that she cuddles while sleeping, and then wind the mobile up and walk out. This reinforcement of her sleep routine will encourage her to resettle herself and go back to sleep.

White noise

White noise can also be used in exactly the same way as a mobile if you would prefer – but use it instead of, rather than as well as, one. Too many cues just become complicated for babies to understand; it is best to keep things simple. You can download white noise apps for most smartphones and tablets, or buy a CD containing various household sounds. Many babies find the sound of the Hoover, a hairdryer, a washing machine and tumble dryer, to name a few, very comforting. These types of noises remind them of the sounds they heard while in the womb. They will have been used to a fair amount of noise on a constant basis while inside you, as they hear your heart beating, your blood rushing around your body and all of the voices on the outside that have become amplified, as they float around cocooned in your tummy.

Once babies are born and put down to sleep in a quiet environment, they can become quite unsettled with the lack of noise. Playing white noise sounds when you are trying to encourage your baby to settle to sleep will sound very familiar to her and be a comforting presence. The sounds will reassure her and help her to relax enough to doze off.

The most important thing to remember when using white noise or a mobile as a cue to encourage your baby to go to sleep is to only play it for a 10-minute period as a maximum, or until your baby has fallen asleep if she has been very unsettled when you attempt to turn it off. If you let it play continuously as she sleeps and she hears it when she wakes up again, as she inevitably will, then it cannot be used as a cue or sleep association.

Switch the white noise or her mobile on as the final thing you do before walking out of the room. If it does not have the ability to turn off automatically, then go in once your baby has settled to sleep and switch it off. In the case of a musical mobile that winds up, most of these stop automatically once the turns have been completed.

If she begins crying immediately after the mobile or white noise has stopped on its own, then allow her five minutes or so to settle herself. She should 'cry down' fairly quickly – this method is explained in more detail in the cry-it-out section below. Her crying will just be her initial frustration that the noise has stopped. However, if she seems to be getting louder and more cross, rather than settling, then go in and check on her after five minutes. Pick her up to calm her down and check that she hasn't got any wind by patting her back. If, again, she is fine and seems to relax into you sleepily then put her down in the basket or cot again, put the mobile or white noise on again and walk out of the room. This extra repetition is sometimes all that is needed to encourage her to settle to sleep. If she doesn't, then look to the other possible causes of her crying.

Cry-it-out or controlled crying

This is a subject open to much debate among parents who already have babies and young children. A lot of the negativity surrounding this method would be reversed or understood if people took the time to research exactly what is involved and when this method is most effective.

The cry-it-out or controlled-crying method is about responding to your baby's needs rather than simply giving in to her wants. It involves understanding your baby's cries and knowing when she genuinely needs you to go to her, and her being sure that you will respond to her when she is genuinely distressed. It is *not*, as some people seem to think, putting her in her cot to cry herself to sleep while you go downstairs with a nice cup of tea and turn the TV volume up loud so you can't hear her crying.

Babies don't naturally fall into a good feeding and sleep routine themselves. It is the parents' job to steer them gently in the right direction and encourage good habits from a very young age. If you do this then your baby's ability to self-soothe and settle to sleep will be much better.

It is important that you respond to her cries quickly while she is under the age of four weeks. After this age you will notice that she is beginning to understand her routine a bit more and will naturally show signs of tiredness and hunger at the usual daily times you have established. You will probably also notice that she is more alert and doesn't necessarily fall asleep in your arms easily or at the end of a feed as before. She may still seem wide-awake as you move towards the naptimes that have been established.

This is the age at which it is important to begin to introduce the sleep cues described previously if you haven't already. This will help her to understand when it is time to sleep. From the age of five to six weeks she will be old enough and feel secure and confident enough to be able to self-soothe after a few minutes of crying, when it is time for her day naps.

Research into sleep training

A study has found that using 'behavioural training' to get babies to sleep, such as leaving them to cry, or practising 'controlled crying' doesn't harm them emotionally or developmentally in the long term.

The findings, which were published by an Australian research team in the journal **Pediatrics**, discovered that out of 225 six-year-olds, those who had undergone 'sleep training' as infants were no different in terms of emotional health from those who did not.

The study is a continuation of some earlier research published in 2007, which concluded that children and their parents benefited when babies were taught to settle themselves to sleep via behavioural techniques. Concerns have previously been raised by medics and parents that leaving a baby to cry, or using other techniques to get them to settle, could have an effect on their emotional development, and their long-term mental health and ability to deal with stress, as well as their relationship with their parents.

The lead author of the latest report, Anna Price, said her team from the Royal Children's Hospital in Victoria, Australia, wanted to see if the benefits were really long lasting and if there were any long-term effects. She and her fellow researchers used the same children and parents they monitored for the 2007 study to answer their questions. In the original study 326 children who were problem sleepers underwent various sleep-encouraging techniques with the help of nurses. At the end of the study, researchers found certain methods like 'controlled comforting' and 'camping out' (where a parent slowly leaves the room over a period of time) improved the infants' sleep and the mothers' depression. The researchers could not find any differences when it came to the children's emotions, conduct or stress, and in the parents they did not find a difference between those who had tried sleep training and those who did not when it came to rates of anxiety or stress. They also did not find any differences in the bond between parent and child between the two groups.

Anna Price told Reuters Health that results show that sleep techniques are safe for children and that it addresses any fears about possible harm 'quite conclusively'.

Below I have described how to teach your baby to settle herself from the age of six weeks onwards using the controlled and timed comforting technique. This explains how to encourage her to settle without help, but when you need to respond to her if she is having difficulty settling.

- Either swaddle your baby fully or half-swaddle her in her cot or Moses basket. If your baby has been happy to be half-swaddled for a while during her day and night sleeps, then this is also a very good age to get her used to a grobag or sleeping bag for her sleep times. It is advisable to do this transition gradually. Put her in her grobag during her day sleeps first and then progress to her evening and full night-time sleep if she continues to sleep well during her day naps.
- Give her a muslin or comfort toy to hold, as described earlier, once she has her hands free from a swaddle.

- Place her in her preferred sleeping position in the Moses basket or cot.
- Close the blind and curtains to ensure the room is as dark as possible.
- Wind up her mobile, or switch on her white noise sounds and say 'night-night' before walking out of the room, closing the door and switching any light off as you go.

Your baby may not cry initially as you walk out of the room. The white noise or cot mobile music will provide a good distraction for her to begin with at least.

Depending on whether her sleep noise cue switches off automatically or not, she is most likely to begin crying a few minutes after you have left the room or when the music stops.

If this is the case then it is okay to let her cry for a few minutes, particularly if she is just whimpering every now and then and not actually crying continuously. You may find that her cries simply stop after a few minutes and she settles herself to sleep.

However, if her cries seem to be increasing rather than tailing off then you need to go in to see what is wrong.

Pick her up and put her over your shoulder. Pat her back to check for wind and at the same time say 'shhh, shhh'. (See the pat-and-shhh technique, page 199.) Once she seems calm and relaxed in your arms and has possibly burped, which could have been the cause of her increasing crying, put her down again, re-swaddle if needed and wind the mobile up or switch the white noise back on as you walk out of the room.

The process of her 'crying down', as it is known, should never take any longer than 10 minutes from the point that she starts crying to the point at which she stops and settles to sleep. It is very important to listen to the length of time that the pause between cries lasts each time. This is your biggest indicator as to whether she will be able to settle herself. If you listen, and she begins whimpering, but after a few minutes the gaps between each noise she makes is increasing and the crying bouts last for a shorter time, then wait another couple of minutes before deciding to go in. This 'crying down', where the crying bouts shorten and the quiet periods lengthen, means that she is gradually settling herself. If she needs you to go in, then her crying will increase rather than decrease, or remain continuous.

> **Tip**
> It is very important to remember that this 10-minute crying-down period restarts each time that you have to go in and resettle her.

If you have had to go in and check for wind and resettle her, then one of two things will happen. She will either settle down immediately, particularly if it was wind that was bothering her and you managed to relieve her of it, or she will get very angry the second time that you put her back down and walk out of the room, and will begin yelling immediately.

This is a very normal reaction and her cry will be a very loud, furious, almost continuous, cry with her barely pausing for breath, and it will last for around two minutes. At the two-to-three-minute point you should begin to hear your first short pause between her cries. Each time the crying resumes it will still be very loud and angry, but, as the minutes tick along, the gaps between her cries will become longer and her bouts of crying much shorter. This will tell you that she has begun to 'cry down'. By the 10-minute mark she should have stopped or be almost at the point of stopping and going to sleep. As long as the gaps continue to get longer and the bursts of crying shorter, then she definitely WILL settle herself to sleep alone.

Those initial two minutes can feel and seem like a lifetime as you listen to her cry – I used to try to busy myself with quickly hanging the washing out or something, while she got that initial angry cry out of her system. As a parent, we never want to hear our children upset or crying as it pulls at our heartstrings. However, the process of teaching them to settle themselves means that in the short term a bit of crying out is necessary to get the long-term result. This does your baby no harm at all socially, emotionally or physically, as studies have proved. As long as you respond to her with love and affection at times when she genuinely needs it, then she will always feel secure and confident. Your instinct as a parent will play a big part in knowing when these times are.

If her crying changes again, and her crying periods increase and the gaps decrease, then you need to go in and repeat the settling process. Go into her room. First of all, just try the pat-and-shhh technique as she is lying in her Moses basket or cot. If she doesn't calm down and continues to cry, then pick her up and check for wind again by placing her over your shoulder. It also may be worth checking her nappy to see if she is soiled. Once she is relaxed and settled over your shoulder again then put her back down. Continue with the pat-and-shhh technique if needed.

The cry-it-out method is a form of self-settling when your baby is young to teach her how to fall asleep on her own using sleep associations such as white noise and mobiles, with controlled comforting when needed. It will benefit her greatly to learn how to self-settle, and as long as you are consistent then she will quickly develop the ability to go to sleep without help from you. She will also understand that when she is genuinely upset, due to wind or any other problem, she won't be ignored and you will go and comfort her.

Over the following weeks after beginning the cry-it-out method and encouraging your baby to self-settle as much as possible, she will soon stop crying when you put her down, and begin to settle by chatting to herself, before drifting off to sleep.

An important part of the self-settling technique also relies on you controlling her wake-up time effectively. The ideal scenario is that you will be the one to go in and wake her up. This should be done by entering the room she is sleeping in and opening the curtains, or switching the light on, as you chat to her. You can greet her by saying, 'Good morning/afternoon – it's time to wake up,' or something similar. Call her name to wake her from her dozy, sleepy state. Allow her to wake up gradually as you chat to her and once she opens her eyes, and possibly smiles at you in response – which is always a lovely greeting – you can pick her up.

If you hear her shuffling around and beginning to wake up and it is around the time you would usually wake her up anyway, then go in and open the curtains in the same way, before she begins to cry.

The most crucial part of the waking-up process from the age of six weeks onwards is that you always try to get to your baby *before* she starts crying. Quite simply, this prevents her associating crying with someone getting her up out of bed. If you always wait until she cries during her daytime naps before going in to get her up, then she will always wake up crying, as she will think that this is the right thing to do to get your attention. As she gets older and begins to self-settle herself to sleep from awake, with a minimal amount of crying or even none at all, she will also start to wake up cooing and chatting. You will encourage her to always wake up in this way, if you ensure that you always go in and get her up while she is still chatty and happy. Sticking to this simple rule will go a very long way to encouraging good long-term sleeping habits. It is fine to let her coo and chat for five to ten minutes, or even longer as she gets older, before you go in and get her up. Make sure you are fully aware of when her chatting begins to turn into a frustrated noise, and go in and do your usual wake-up routine of opening the curtains, and chatting to her before she starts to cry.

In my experience the parents, including myself, that have stuck to this simple rule have babies that settle to sleep very easily, and also wake up in a very cheerful happy mood every time they go to sleep, right into toddlerhood. It will also give you a major insight into when there is a problem that needs your attention. If it is unusual for your baby to cry when you put her down to sleep, or if she wakes up crying, then it can indicate a problem. Teething, illnesses or having a wet or soiled nappy are just some of the examples of things that can upset your baby and prevent her from settling as well as she usually would.

Controlled and timed comforting technique

This method is very effective for babies and parents who prefer not to do the full cry-it-out method, although with some babies who are in particularly bad habits that is sometimes the only option. It involves going in to comfort and reassure your baby after a timed period, but then leaving the room again to encourage self-settling.

- *You wind your baby down as you usually would with a calm environment, story and feed etc.*
- *Put her down in the cot, give her any comforter she is used to (teddy, muslin, etc.) and wind up her mobile or switch her white noise cue device on.*
- *Use the pat-and-shhh technique for 15–30 seconds. With an older baby who can move around the cot and try to sit or stand you need to be quite firm. Lie her on her tummy and hold her there firmly with one hand while patting her bottom with the other hand in a heartbeat rhythm and say 'shhh' loudly. If she tries to fight you and struggle away from your pat and shhh then stop doing it. Trust your instinct as to when to leave the room.*
- *If your baby is old enough to get up and stand and does this as you leave the room, just ignore it and carry on going out.*
- *The idea now is to return after two minutes and then add two minutes each time to the last time you went in.*
- *Go back in after two minutes. Lie her down again on her tummy and pat and shhh for 15–30 seconds and then leave again. Try to avoid making any eye contact.*

- *Wait for four minutes then go in and repeat the pat and shhh, then leave the room.*
- *Wait for six minutes, then repeat.*
- *Wait for eight minutes then repeat, then ten minutes.*
- *If you get to the 10-minute mark then you don't need to increase the gaps any longer. Stick to 10-minute intervals thereafter.*

You need to listen for gaps and pauses in her crying as described in the controlled-crying section. This will be the start of the 'crying down' period and her settling herself to sleep. You will usually begin to hear the pauses around the six-to-eight minute wait mark. Once you start hearing pauses, particularly if it is just before you are due to go in again, then it is worth waiting a little longer before going in. If the pauses continue to become longer and she is crying for shorter periods then you may not need to go in again at all. Use your instinct to judge this, as going in just as she is beginning to settle, may add 'fuel to her fire' and seeing you again may mean it takes her a longer time to resettle.

If the gaps in her crying begin to increase again then go in and repeat the pat-and-shhh technique and add another two minutes to the time you got up to when you leave the room.

In my experience, all babies have usually settled to sleep or are having long pauses between cries and almost asleep by the 10-minute wait mark, although with an older baby you may go into the first or even second 10-minute mark on your first session of timed comforting.

This method is very effective for babies who have been used to being fed, cuddled or rocked to sleep, or relying on a dummy and are waking frequently at night. The best time to start implementing this method is at the 7 p.m. bedtime sleep. Once she settles the first time you use the above method, then repeat it each time she wakes in the night and then also for all naps at the suggested times for her age.

Combine the settling technique with the wake-up routine, so that she begins to learn to settle to sleep and wake up without crying.

The timed/controlled comforting method will also work for babies who are relying on a pat or shhh to get them to sleep and wake frequently for that to resettle them to sleep in the night. Use the method as described above but when you go in the room each time only pat and shhh for 10–20 seconds as a maximum. This will stop her going completely off to sleep as you pat and teach her how to settle herself.

Many parents find the controlled timed comforting technique preferable to the full controlled crying method. The full controlled crying method should only be attempted once a baby is over six months.

Early-morning waking

If your baby has been previously sleeping well until 7 a.m. or later and begins waking early, it could be due to any of the following reasons:

- **Too cold**: Ensure she has enough layers of clothing. Even in the summer months when the daytime temperature is particularly hot, the night-time temperature always drops to its lowest point between 4 and 7 a.m. If your baby doesn't have enough layers on or has kicked her blankets off, then she is very likely to wake up cold, particularly during that period of the night when she will be in her lightest sleep. It is good to get her used to a sleeping bag or grobag from an early age if possible. They can be bought in various tog ratings suitable for summer or winter use and help to keep your baby's temperature at a constant level, and prevent her waking up feeling cold. They are also a much safer option than blankets, particularly once your baby begins to roll and crawl.

- **Hungry:** If you haven't begun weaning yet and your baby begins to wake in the night after previously dropping the night feed and sleeping well, then she could be waking due to hunger. Rather than resorting to reintroducing her night feed, I would advise that you increase all of her day feeds until you decide that the time is right to wean her. You should also increase the 10–11 p.m. feed up to a maximum of 9fl oz (260ml) if needed. This can then be reduced as described in Chapter 4, once weaning has been established.

- **Soiled or wet nappy:** If your baby is regularly waking up wet and soaked through to the bedcovers in the early hours of the morning, then you can put two nappies on her, one on top of the other, when you put her to bed (see page 153). You don't need to buy a different size, two of the same size works just fine. Adding the extra nappy over the top of the first one acts as a safety net to catch any excess wee. More often than not the top nappy will still be dry when you take it off in the morning and it can then be used as her first nappy of the day, so that you are not using any more nappies than you need.

  If she is waking up with a soiled nappy then the best thing you can do is to change her quickly, using a minimum amount of light, and try to resettle her back to sleep. If she has already been weaned, then cutting protein out of her diet at teatime will change her bowel habits and mean she is much less likely to continue to wake with a soiled nappy. Any kind of meat-based meal should be given at lunchtime, as this tends to be what causes a soiled nappy in the early morning if given at teatime. Her tea should be a meal consisting of purely vegetables or lentils or a dairy-based meal with no meat involved.

- **Teething:** If your baby is already showing some of the signs of teething (discussed in more detail in Chapter 7) during the daytime, then it is possible any night waking could also be due to teething pain, when she comes into a light sleep.

With teething pain a baby can end up crying inconsolably. No amount of soothing or cuddling seems to help ease the crying, and it will continue until you can give her some form of teething treatment to ease the pain. Try Anbesol liquid first, which can be bought from pharmacies and some major supermarkets. I have found this product to be the best by far for relieving teething pain as it contains an anaesthetic and antiseptic solution to give immediate relief. I would suggest applying that at night-time and, after a cuddle to soothe your baby, put her back down again in her cot to see if she will settle back to sleep. If she continues to cry and doesn't seem to be moving towards crying down and going back to sleep, then it is more likely that the pain is more severe and you need to give her a paracetamol or Nurofen dose of medicine. In my experience, an ibruprofen-based medicine is more effective in relieving teething pain. If you do need to give either of these (providing your baby is over 12 weeks), then you will also need to sit with her for 20 minutes or so. This is how long the medicine takes to begin giving some pain relief. Sit in a chair in the nursery, where possible, with only low lighting, rather than bringing her out of the room, so that she doesn't get too stimulated. Once the 20-minute mark has passed then you can attempt to put her back in her cot. Go through your usual bedtime process of placing her to sleep in her preferred position, giving her a muslin or comfort toy to cuddle, and winding the mobile up or switching on her white noise before you go out.

Once you have eliminated any pain and made sure that nothing else is upsetting her and causing her early-morning waking, then she should be able to self-settle herself to sleep with a very short cry-it-out or controlled comforting period.

Top tip

If your baby is regularly waking early in the morning and none of the above seem to be the cause, then you could try waking her more fully and keeping her awake for a bit longer during the 10–11 p.m. feed. If she has been sleeping well from 7 p.m. up until this feed and having to be woken and then still remains sleepy during the feed, then this could be the reason she is waking early.

Wake her fully at this feed and bring her downstairs. Have the TV on and chat to her to wake her up properly. Change her nappy and begin the feed once she has been fully awake for a minimum of 15 minutes. Let her have the first half of her bottle-feed or breastfeed downstairs. Once you have winded her then you can continue the second part of the feed back in her room with the lights low and with no stimulation. This will encourage her to drift back off to sleep more easily at the end of the feed. By waking her fully and making the feed last a bit longer by splitting it, then she should sleep better, without the usual early-morning waking.

Sleep problems or associations in older babies

Below I have described some of the most common sleep problems or associations that are formed when no routine is established from an early age, and how to solve them.

Being fed to sleep

This is a particularly common habit for breastfed babies to develop. When a baby is young, they naturally fall asleep at the breast as it is so comforting for them. It can be very easy for mothers to fall into the habit of thinking that their babies must be full and have had enough milk when they fall asleep at the breast. In reality, the baby will not have fed for long enough to sustain herself for any decent stretch of time and will wake again a short time later, rooting around for the breast again. Very quickly a vicious circle of snack feeding develops. The baby will be genuinely hungry through not taking enough of the hind milk, so will need to feed again. However, she will also get used to the habit of always being fed back to sleep, particularly at night-time. She will then begin to rely on this sleep association of being fed to resettle herself every time. Pretty soon the mother becomes exhausted from the baby's constant demands, and the baby isn't very happy either.

Solution

You need to encourage your baby to take full breastfeeds on a regular basis during the daytime. If she begins to fall asleep at the breast and stops feeding then try to stimulate her to continue by tickling her, or stroking her cheek and talking to her as you feed to wake her up. If she has fallen completely asleep, but hasn't spent an adequate amount of time on the breast to have reached the important hind milk, then you need to remove her from the breast and wake her up again fully. This can be done by undressing her or changing her nappy. If she is bottle-fed and has also resorted to this sleepy snack feeding you can also use these methods to wake her up and encourage her to finish a full feed. Establish a regular feeding pattern during the daytime, as described in Chapter 4. Once you baby is feeding regularly during the day and encouraged to wait three to four hours between feeds, her night-time waking will improve dramatically. Don't allow her to have her bottle in the cot to drink; she will be relying on this to get herself to sleep. Get her into the habit of drinking her milk downstairs, or if you prefer her to have it in the nursery then have her sitting on your lap to drink it, rather than lying in her cot alone.

You can cuddle her to a drowsy state rather than feed her to sleep to help break the cycle, although establishing a feeding routine will have the biggest impact. Progress the sleep routine by putting your baby down to sleep drowsy and use the pat-and-shhh technique to help settle her to sleep.

It really depends on the type of baby you have, as different methods work better for different babies when you try to introduce them to an older baby or child.

If the pat-and-shhh technique just seems to wind her up, then you can try sitting next to her cot until she calms down. If she is old enough to move around and pull herself to standing then you should get up and lie her back down each time she stands up. The trick is to stay very calm, avoid any eye contact and each time you lie her back down just say, 'it's night-night-time,' or something similar that you prefer to repeat. You should then sit back down next to the cot, without looking at her. Eventually she will realise that she is not getting any attention from you and will stay lying down and settle to sleep.

Another option is to use the controlled and timed comforting method. This technique is the most effective in encouraging babies to settle themselves to sleep who have previously been relying on the breast as a form of comfort, and it is my preferred method that I suggest to the many mums that email me daily. It means you are still able to comfort and reassure, but you are also encouraging your baby to learn to settle to sleep without the breast as a sleep prop. It is also one step before the full cry-it-out method that every parent would prefer to avoid. Combining the timed comforting method with the wake-up routine will ensure this method works quickly and with the minimum amount of crying.

The final option, if you have tried everything else, is the cry-it-out method. Depending on the age of your baby and how bad the habit has become, then it will take a much longer cry-it-out period of time. Use the process described earlier on in the chapter. The key, as always, is to listen for the gaps between cries. The first initial bout of crying will always be very furious, angry crying with barely any pauses. Once you begin to get gaps then, as long as they continue to increase and the crying bouts lessen, she should settle herself to sleep. Remember that each time you have to go in and calm her down then your cry-it-out time technically restarts.

With some babies it can reach a stage where you need to leave them for a longer period of time to cry to break the habit. I always hate suggesting it to parents – as a mother myself I know how tough it is having to listen to your baby cry at all – but if very bad habits have been formed then sometimes it is the final and only option. If you do have to resort to the full controlled-crying method then the maximum amount of time it takes is five nights of consistency. As long as you are sure your baby is well and you have satisfied yourself that she is not teething, hungry, cold, hot or has a soiled nappy, then it is perfectly safe to leave her to cry it out for a longer period of time.

Being cuddled or rocked to sleep

Again, this is a very easy habit to slip into. Babies are so very cuddly and as a parent you never seem to get enough of having a little snuggle together – it's lovely for both of you. However, as your baby gets older she will begin to rely on always being cuddled to sleep if she has never been put down for a nap awake to learn to settle herself, or always been in the car or pushchair to go to sleep. In the beginning it never seems to be a big issue, but the older she gets she will then start to wake regularly during the night, because she has never learned to settle herself. This can happen five to ten times per night in some cases, every time she comes into a light sleep and realises she is not in your arms any more.

Solution

The solution is to use some or all of the same methods described above to solve the feeding-to-sleep issue.

- Establish a feeding routine during the daytime.
- Begin to try to put your baby down drowsy rather than completely asleep.
- Use the pat-and-shhh technique, sitting next to the cot method, controlled and timed comforting method, or cry-it-out method

to encourage your baby to begin to learn how to self-settle. Ensure you have read the sleep structure advised for babies of varying ages described earlier on in this chapter, so that you know roughly how much and when she should be sleeping during the daytime.

Sleeping in parents' bed: co-sleeping

At certain points co-sleeping is a very common thing for many parents to do with their baby, occasionally at least, in the early days and weeks. It is only when this is continued past the age of 10–12 weeks and is a regular nightly occurrence that a baby begins to rely on the comfort of having a parent beside them all the time. To begin with it can work very well for some parents and ensures that everybody gets a good night's sleep. However, for many, it eventually becomes more of a problem as the baby grows bigger and begins to wake frequently at night each time she enters a light sleep and then becomes more difficult to settle down. Parents can then resort to feeding the baby back to sleep, which creates another problem, and the night waking continues to the point where everybody is exhausted and things need to change.

Solution

There is no easy solution to breaking this habit. If your baby has been sleeping with you every night over a long period of time, then to go from that to sleeping alone will be a big change for her. You will need to follow the steps below to make the change to her learning to sleep alone in her own cot or bed.

- Ensure her feeding and sleep is structured during the day. This will give you peace of mind that she is definitely not hungry when she cries at night. Ensuring that she also has regular naps during the day means she will not be so overtired when it is time to settle her down to sleep. This may take you a few days to establish well. During this time, allow her to take her naps wherever she is used to having them and get her to sleep in the usual way too – even if that means that you have to settle her in some way.

- Once her feeding and daytime sleeps have been established then you can work on the evening and night-time routine. I would suggest starting her off in her cot in her own room when you put her down at 7 p.m. for her evening sleep. Breast- or bottle-feed her as you normally would and put her down in her cot to sleep. If you haven't already established any good sleep associations, like her having a muslin or comfort toy to hold and listening to a sleep cue, like a mobile or white noise CD to settle, then now is also the time to start this.

- Place her in the cot with a muslin or comfort toy. Wind her mobile up or switch on the white noise CD and walk out of the room, turning the light off as you go and say 'night-night'.

- It is highly likely she will cry very angrily. In my experience the timed comforting is the most effective method to use to encourage your baby to self settle in their own cot. Combined with the wake-up routine described earlier, your baby will settle down very quickly and sleep for much longer periods at night once she has the ability to self settle without relying on your presence.

- If you would prefer then you can try sitting next to her cot as a way to reassure her, while she settles to sleep. Each time she stands up, then you need to lie her back down calmly and repeat 'night-night', and then sit back down again next to the cot. Some parents find doing this makes the transition for their baby and themselves much easier. However, for some babies having you sit next to the cot but not actually pick them up is too distressing and makes the whole settling process much harder.

You can then progress to the cry-it-out method if you need to at a later stage, if you don't feel the other methods are working; it will be up to you to gauge what works for you and your baby.

CASE STUDY: The cry-it-out method in action

Natalie called me when her baby girl Isabel was eight months old. She was sleeping in their bed every night and was waking five to ten times per night to be resettled with a cuddle or pat. Both parents were exhausted and their marriage was beginning to suffer terribly from the strain. Isabel was very grumpy during the daytimes, due to poor sleeping patterns, and during the day had only ever slept in the pushchair or car seat for short naps. It was obvious that she had never learned how to settle herself, so that was going to be our big hurdle.

I advised Natalie that she needed to establish a daytime feeding and sleep routine first of all, which she began to do over the next few days. Once that was done, I gave Natalie two options. As Isabel had never had to settle herself to sleep at all from awake, it was going to be a big change for her. I advised her to attempt to settle Isabel in her cot that night for her 7 p.m. bedtime, but that Natalie could stay in the room in the dark and sit next to the cot with her for reassurance. Each time Isabel sat or stood up, she was to lie her back down again calmly and say, 'night-night-time,' and then resume her sitting position on the floor. Once she had settled to sleep, then Natalie could creep out of the room. If she woke again, then she should go back in and repeat the same process again.

I did also warn her that with some babies this can make them even more frustrated and, if after a couple of nights of this it didn't seem to be working, then we may have to resort to the cry-it-out method to break the habit.

Natalie called me the next day and said that she thought Isabel just got more irate with having her sit there but not picking her up and bring her into their bed, so she would rather just go ahead and try the cry-it-out method. I explained it was going to be awful for everyone concerned, but if she stuck with the simple rules I gave her, then within three to five nights Isabel would be settling herself to sleep all the time without too much fuss. She agreed that she was ready to try anything, as the whole family couldn't continue with the way things were.

The rules to follow were:

- *At no point should Isabel be brought into her parents' bed again. If Natalie thought she was having difficulty settling at any point, she was to* go into her room to reassure her but not bring her out of the room. She could pick her up to calm her down, pat her or give her a short cuddle in the chair in the nursery, but Isabel needed to learn to understand that her parents' bed was no longer an option. I told Natalie if she stuck to this rule then, although the first couple of nights would be very tough, Isabel would quickly get the idea and settle down.

• I advised Natalie to establish a sleep cue like a mobile or CD that she could always use when putting Isabel down to sleep. She said there was a mobile above Isabel's cot but they didn't always use it. I told her that it would be a good idea to begin winding this up every time she put Isabel down and repeating 'night-night' before leaving her to settle. If at any point she needed to go in and resettle Isabel then the mobile should be wound up again before leaving the room to indicate to Isabel that it was still sleep time.

The first night Natalie put Isabel down at 7:30 p.m. She had been very happy all day and fed and slept very well, which had now been established as a good routine. She cried as soon as Natalie left the room and was very angry for the first 10 minutes. Natalie had a camera baby monitor so she could see her on the monitor and knew that she was safe. Ten minutes in and Natalie saw on the monitor that she had made herself sick in the cot. I told her this was very normal for some babies and she should go into her room and clean Isabel and the cot as quickly as possible. She should avoid talking to her but could say 'shhh, shhh' to calm her if she was still crying, avoiding eye contact as much as possible, and then put her back down into her cot again. The mobile should again be wound up and Natalie should leave her to settle. After another 10-minute period of crying, Isabel again made herself sick. Natalie went in again, cleaned her up and resettled her in her cot. This time, after another 10 minutes of crying, Isabel did her first longer pause between crying bouts. She continued to leave pauses between crying over the next half an hour, with the pauses gradually becoming longer and the crying bursts shorter. Although listening to the crying was very tough for her parents, hearing the pauses gave them some reassurance that they were heading in the right direction and she was settling. If her crying did begin to increase again then I told them that this would indicate a problem and they would have to go in. Isabel's crying continued to decrease until she finally went quiet and settled herself to sleep at 9 p.m. Her parents were amazed – she had never done this on her own in eight months. Knowing that she had settled herself also gave them the confidence to stick with this method and know that it was the right way to go to solve Isabel's bad sleeping habits.

I advised her parents that if Isabel woke in the night, they should go in, pick her up and give her a cuddle and then, once calm, put her back down with her comfort toy, wind the mobile up and walk out, saying, 'night-night,' and leave her to settle herself again in the same way.

Another crucial part of encouraging a baby to self-settle is you being the one to control the wake-up time. I advised Natalie that she needed to try to get into Isabel's room in the morning and be the one to wake her up if possible, as this would really help her ability to settle better and wake up in a happy chatty mood, long term, rather than associating crying with getting up. Natalie set her alarm for 6 a.m. but was expecting Isabel to wake her long before that and have to do the controlled crying again.

Much to her parents' surprise and delight, Isabel slept straight through the night without a peep for the first time! Natalie was woken by her alarm at 6 a.m. and turned over to look at the video monitor and find Isabel still sound asleep. She continued to watch on tenterhooks until 6:45 a.m. when Isabel began to shuffle around and stir. At that point, Natalie went into her room, opened the curtains and said, 'Good morning,' and was greeted with a lovely smile.

That evening at 7 p.m. when Isabel was put to bed, she settled much better. There were no sickness episodes and, after a much shorter crying-down period over 45 minutes, she was asleep by 8 p.m. Again, she slept through the night and Natalie was able to go in and wake her around 7 a.m. in the morning. By the third night Isabel's crying period decreased dramatically and after only a 10-minute total crying-down period she settled herself to sleep and again slept all night without a peep. Isabel continued to sleep well on a regular basis after this, with the exception of teething episodes and illnesses making her unsettled on occasions. However, because she was now in an established routine, Natalie was able to gauge when *something was actually wrong with her because it was now unusual for her to be upset and unsettled when going to bed. Her parents found it much easier to meet Isabel's needs now that she had an established sleeping routine, and at almost two years old she continues to settle herself and sleep very well in her own bed.*

Attachment to a dummy

Many parents find the use of a dummy during the early days and weeks very helpful in establishing a feeding routine. I have always positively encouraged use of them for this reason. Newborn babies tend to want to suck frequently as a form of comfort. Making use of a dummy prevents the risk of falling into the habit of snack feeding a baby, which can lead to all sorts of wind-related problems, colic and reflux. If a dummy is used in the right way then your baby will not become dependent on it. However, if it is frequently given to get her off to sleep and she is left to continue sucking it while asleep, then she will very quickly become reliant on the use of it to get herself to sleep all of the time. This is even more likely if you continue to use it once she is over the age of 12 weeks. To begin with, it may not seem like she is attached to it. Eventually she will get to the point of looking for the dummy to be put back into her mouth every time she comes into a light sleep in the middle of the night. The fact that this can happen between five to ten times per night, means that each time she will cry and wake you up to ask for the dummy again. This dummy dependency with the frequent night waking generally happens between six and twelve months of age.

Solution

At the point you realise that she is dependent on the dummy you have two choices. The first is that you continue to get up and replace the dummy until she gets to the age where she can move around the cot and find a carefully placed one herself.

The second option is that you stop use of the dummy altogether. Unfortunately the only way to do this is to go 'cold turkey'. The best time to start it is when it is time to put her down for her evening sleep at 7 p.m. If she doesn't already use any other form of comforter like a muslin or tag toy then now is the time to introduce one as a replacement for her dummy. You should also introduce use of a cot mobile or white noise CD as a sleep cue, as described earlier.

The timed comforting method should be used, which has been described previously (see page 218) to encourage her to settle without using the dummy.

It is essential that, once you decide to stop using the dummy, you throw them all away so that you are not tempted to give in and let her have it once she has been crying for a while. This would be the worst thing you could do, as it sends her the message that if she cries for long enough you will always give in and allow her to have what she wants in the end.

Rolling on to her tummy or standing up in the cot and getting 'stuck'

Many babies learn to roll over on to their front before they learn to roll back again. Once they can do this they frequently roll over but can get very frustrated at not being able to roll back again, and will cry until helped on to their back again. This can happen during the night too and parents are woken up by their baby crying to be rolled on to their back again. Some babies actually prefer tummy sleeping and are happy to stay sleeping on their front once they reach the rolling stage and won't cry to be rolled back. If your baby is one of these then it is perfectly safe to leave her to sleep on her tummy if that is the sleeping position she prefers. If she is old enough and strong enough to roll then she is also physically able to hold her head and neck up and away from the mattress, so the risk of cot death dramatically reduces anyway.

As your baby gets older, she may also learn how to pull herself to standing but, again, doesn't always learn how to sit back down again immediately, so will cry for help to lie her back down.

Solution

You can try tucking her sleeping bag down into the mattress to prevent her rolling over as easily when in her cot if she is frequently doing this. The best solution for both the rolling-over and standing-up issues is to teach her to roll back and sit herself down again. Practise teaching her how to do this repeatedly in the daytime during play and she will soon learn how to do the reverse of what she has already learned. Patience and perseverance, as always, will get you there! Once she can roll back over and sit herself down from standing she will be able to resettle herself in the cot without needing your help.

Until she gets to this stage then the best method to use would be the controlled and timed comfort method described previously.

Top tips to remember – a summary so far

- If breastfeeding, it is important to encourage your baby to feed for long enough on one side to reach the important hind milk. This will prevent her snack feeding, which can lead to excess wind and colic. If bottle-feeding, try to stick to three-to-four-hourly feeding during the day, again to prevent the problems that snack feeding causes. Try increasing her bottle teat size if she is very slow to feed or not taking a lot at each feed but still seems hungry before the next feed.
- Bottles should be sterilised until your baby is 12 months old.
- Always remove your baby's bib before putting her down to sleep. It is very dangerous for her to sleep wearing it as she is at risk of being strangled by it as she moves her head around in her sleep.
- Remember the two-hour rule where sleep is concerned in the first eight to ten weeks. Your baby must be down and asleep within two hours of the last time that she woke up, to prevent overtiredness. Once over this age she will begin to be able to manage to stay awake for a slightly longer period of time than this.

- Once you begin to encourage her to self-settle over the age of six weeks it is important that you go to her when she wakes up in the morning as much as possible *before* she begins to get upset and cry. This will help her to continue to wake happy and be content to play and chat when settling to sleep too.

- Cow's milk can be given in food from the age of six to seven months, but only given to drink when your baby is over 12 months old.

- Spending extra time making sure your baby is well winded at the last feed of the evening (10:30 p.m. feed) will mean she is more likely to sleep better over the core hours of the night, rather than being unsettled and waking repeatedly because of excess wind.

- Like us, babies vary in how hungry they are at different times of the day and even from one day to the next. Try not to worry if she seems to want to drink less on particular days. As long as she seems well and you don't resort to snack feeding, or reintroducing a night feed, her appetite will come back and she's bound to then make up for what she has missed out on by eating more on the following days after that.

- When needed, position her to sleep on her right side, wedged in, using rolled-up towels or blankets to prevent her from rolling on to her back or front. This will be a particularly ideal sleeping position if she suffers from excess wind or reflux and even if she is unwell with a cold or cough.

- Ensure her nappy is done up quite tightly with no gaps down the sides where it sticks together. Make sure the lip that goes round each leg is not tucked in as this can also cause the nappy to leak. A baby boy's penis needs to be pushed gently down before you do the nappy up. Nappy changing takes practice, and you will most likely experience a few entire outfit changes before you get the correct technique that enables the nappy to work effectively and your baby to stay dry.

- Motherhood is not a battle against other mothers. It is your journey with your baby. Don't try to do things with your baby or push her on to the next stage just to keep up with others. She will let you know when she is ready to do everything and make changes.
- There is no way to be a perfect mother, but there are a million ways to be a good one. That is all we can ever strive to be.
- Tomorrow is a new day. No matter how bad a day you have had, then try to get up the next day and forget about the events of the previous one. Babies can have very different moods from one day to the next, just like we as adults do. You will have good days, where she sticks to the routine you have established perfectly. Equally you will have days where nothing seems to go right in terms of her feeding and sleeping. Take each day as it comes, and on the bad days go with the flow a bit more.
- Patience and perseverance will get you to where you want to be in everything you do with your baby. Repeat this to yourself whenever you are feeling stressed and when everything you try doesn't seem to make your baby happy on a particular day. It will give you the strength to carry on!

6
Weaning

There is so much confusion surrounding the subject of when and how to wean your baby. Most parents buy two or three baby books when they are pregnant and I can almost guarantee that they will all differ in their advice on how to wean.

In fact, even NHS guidelines have changed dramatically over the period of time my own three children have been born. In 2002 when my eldest son was born, the advice was to begin weaning no earlier than 16 weeks and to only give dairy and protein from the age of six months. It wasn't unusual at this time for many parents to wean earlier though, from 10–12 weeks. When my second son was born in 2006 the guidelines had changed again, and the NHS was advising mothers to solely breastfeed for six months solid with no supplementing and no solids. If for some reason a mother was unable to breastfeed then the advice was to formula feed their baby up until six months of age. I remember that there was a big push at the time my second child was born towards breastfeeding over bottle-feeding. I know a lot of mums felt a huge amount of pressure to breastfeed by some health professionals at this time, and it was almost frowned upon if they refused to even try and wanted to bottle-feed from the start.

In 2011 when my daughter was born, the guidelines had changed again, and remain the same now in 2014. Current NHS guidelines recommend that a baby should only be fed breast milk or infant formula milk up until the age of six months. Health experts agree that six months is the best age for introducing solids. Before this your baby's digestive system is still developing, and weaning too soon may increase the risk of infections and allergies. They state that if for some reason a parent wants, or needs, to wean their baby earlier, then four months or 17 weeks is the absolute minimum age to introduce solids.

These guidelines apply to full-term babies and do not apply to babies born prematurely. Experts at special care baby charity Bliss recommend that babies who are born prematurely should be weaned between the ages of five and seven months (calculating from your baby's birth date, not the date on which she would have been born if she had reached full term). Very occasionally a prem baby may benefit from being weaned before the age of five months, but this should be discussed with your healthcare team first.

If your baby has particular feeding problems, such as reflux, or a medical condition that makes feeding difficult, the health professionals you see may sometimes – but not always – advise to wean before six months.

The change to six months was introduced after worldwide research endorsed by numerous health bodies, including the Department of Health and the World Health Organization, showed that certain problems could occur. Details are below:

- Your baby's risk of developing allergies and infections may increase and she could go on to have digestive problems and obesity later on in life.
- It may affect the amount of nutrients your baby absorbs if you are breastfeeding.
- Your baby's digestive system and kidneys may not be developed enough to cope safely with solid food.

Foods to avoid before six months old

If your baby is over 17 weeks and you would like to begin weaning, then there are certain foods that you should avoid until she is over six months. They are as follows:

- Dairy products made with cow's milk: yoghurts, cheese, fromage frais, etc.
- Citrus fruits, including fruit juice.
- Foods containing gluten: bread, pasta, rusks, etc.

These are in addition to the other foods listed later, that are to be avoided completely while your baby is less than one year.

Weaning: when, how and what?

When?

There are a few signs to let you know that your baby is physically ready, on top of being the correct age:

1: She can stay in a sitting position and hold her head steady. This can be in a high chair, bouncy chair or Bumbo, not necessarily unaided.
2: She can swallow food. Babies discover their tongue from a young age and love nothing more than poking it out all day long. This is called the extrusion reflex. If she is still doing this a lot then it may be more difficult to get the loaded spoon into her mouth!
3: She has good hand–eye coordination. This is more essential from when you begin offering finger foods, unless you plan to wean using the baby-led weaning method.

Some signs that your baby may display but that do *not* indicate that she is ready for solids based on these reasons alone are:

- Having doubled her birth weight. Many babies have generally done this by six months as a rule of thumb anyway, even most premature babies. Some babies manage to do this long before six months so this is not a reason on which to base the correct time to wean.

- Chewing her hands/fists. All babies do this from around 12 weeks when they develop the hand–eye coordination to be able to purposefully move their hands to their mouths. They are merely exploring their hands, just as they like to explore any rattles or toys that you give them.

- She watches you eat and follows your food. This is just her becoming more interested in anything and everything that moves around her. You wouldn't offer her a cigarette if she was staring intently at somebody who was smoking, would you? So why offer solids for this reason?

- Wanting extra milk. This could be because she's having another growth spurt.

- Begins to wake in the night after previously being a good sleeper. This is more likely to be due to teething pain.

Contrary to popular belief, weaning your baby will not make her sleep any better if you are already having disturbed nights when you get to the weaning stage. It is more likely that your baby has slipped into bad habits if she is not sleeping well at night-time, or that she is not getting an adequate amount of milk or sleep during the day to enable her to be settled at night. If you have picked up this book and already have an older baby who hasn't had a structured feeding and sleeping routine from an early age, then I would advise you to read the chapters on feeding and sleeping before you resort to weaning, particularly if your baby is under six months, and you are hoping weaning will solve all of your baby's sleep issues. It's important that you ensure she is getting enough milk and sleep, and is able to settle herself to sleep, before beginning to wean. Weaning will only cause more problems if you don't, because she may decrease her milk intake, which in turn will affect her sleep even more. A few ounces of milk is more likely to fill her up than a few spoonfuls of purée.

How and what?

If you have read this book and used the advice from day one and your baby follows the same feed and sleep times roughly every day, then the weaning guide times that I will provide will fit in perfectly with what she does on a daily basis.

Once you decide to begin weaning it is very important to remember that milk is still the most important part of your baby's diet, whether it's from the breast or formula in a bottle. Her milk intake should not go down at this stage – introducing solid food is in addition to what she is already taking in.

When you begin weaning you need to offer it to coincide with the milk feeds your baby is already having. The two feeds you should begin giving solids with are the 11 a.m. and the 6 p.m. feeds. It is crucial that you still give her most of her milk feed *before* the solids. You can then offer her a small amount of solids and then the remaining milk feed to 'wash it down'. Later on, as your baby gets older and you introduce protein and bigger meals, her 11 a.m. milk will be reduced and dropped, and this meal pushed closer to 12 p.m. as her lunchtime meal. The 6 p.m. meal will come forward to 4:30/5 p.m., and her bedtime milk will remain but probably at a slightly later time of 6:30/7 p.m.

Breakfast is not usually introduced at this early stage. This meal will come later, once she starts to show signs that milk alone is no longer enough at the 7/8 a.m. feed to be able to get her through happily to the next feed at 11 a.m.

There are two methods available to use when you move your baby on to solids: baby-led weaning and spoon-fed weaning. Details of both are below.

Baby-led weaning

Baby-led weaning (BLW) means simply that you let your baby feed herself by offering a variety of nutritious finger foods suitable for her age. You do not give her any type of purée or spoon-feed her at all. The easiest finger foods for young babies are those that are shaped like a chip, or have a handle, like cooked broccoli. Initially when you first begin weaning your baby will only be able to clasp or grab things in her whole hand or fist, as she won't have developed her pincer grip yet. You need to be careful what foods you introduce to begin with to minimise the risk of choking. Suggested finger foods suitable from six months are:

- Raw slices/chunks of banana, avocado, pears, cucumber (peeled), peaches and melon
- Cooked rice
- Citrus fruits and other fruits such as like kiwi and strawberries
- Baby breadsticks
- Cubes or fingers of bread/toast (can sometimes cause gagging or choking if she puts too much in and it sticks together and becomes gloopy in her mouth)
- Chopped hard-boiled egg

You may choose to start BLW by just offering your baby tasters of the family meal each day. This is fine but ensure the things you give her to try have no added salt or sugar. Ready meals and pasta sauces from jars are not a good idea. Stick to very plain foods with no additives.

At first your baby will just play with the food. She may then begin to grab pieces of food and suck them. Parents who have tried BLW are generally very passionate about its benefits, but they will all admit that the process is very messy, and there is a lot of waste. If most of your baby's food ends up on the floor then there is obviously a limit to the amount of nutrients she will get.

Spoon-led weaning

This is literally as the name suggests – you spoon puréed or mashed food into your baby's mouth. You can gradually make the food you offer on the spoon lumpier and also introduce finger foods too so that your baby has a chance to explore foods with her own hands.

The official advice by the Department of Health, European Union and the World Health Organization, is to give your baby well mashed or puréed foods during the early stages of weaning and then finger foods when you feel they are ready for them.

I wholeheartedly agree with this. Every parent is entitled to their own opinion on which weaning method to use but I found it difficult to comprehend that my baby would get enough nutritious food into her if I allowed her to pick at the food herself from such a young age.

In my opinion it is helpful to wean your baby using both methods. I recommend using the spoon-led weaning method initially, and as your baby becomes more coordinated at picking up various foods you can offer her finger foods at the same time. I have set out my weaning guide below to reflect this method.

For the first few days only offer her baby rice. You can use expressed breast milk or some of the formula out of your baby's made-up bottle to mix with the rice for your baby to eat. Once she gets used to this new idea of taking food from a spoon, you can begin to try her on various fruits and vegetables. I believe that it is very important to offer more vegetable-based, savoury-tasting food in the beginning to prevent your baby getting used to sweet-tasting foods and preferring them to savoury tastes. All babies and children love sweet-tasting things and will show much more enthusiasm for when they are given them to eat. This is a natural reaction and goes on into adulthood, as we can all vouch for!

By introducing more savoury tastes in the beginning your baby will learn to enjoy all foods, sweet and savoury. Don't be put off if she doesn't seem to like a particular food that you try her with over a few days. Try mixing it with various other vegetables at a later stage, or even waiting a few weeks and offering it again. It is very common for babies to dislike a particular taste initially but then eat it quite happily a few weeks later!

Home-cooked purées, as opposed to jars and packet foods, are always going to be healthier for your baby to eat. They also have other advantages:

- They are less expensive to buy and you can make larger quantities of them in the long term.
- It puts you in complete control of what your baby is eating.

Although I would highly recommend making the majority of your baby's food yourself, it is advisable to feed your baby the odd jar. This is so that you know she will eat them if you ever need her to for any reason: days out etc. I found that the fruit purées that you can buy in the supermarkets are great to use as pudding as your baby gets older too, especially as it means you can allow your baby to experience fruits that you may not necessarily buy at the supermarket to purée and freeze.

Equipment and preparation

Below is a list of items and equipment you will need to begin weaning:

- Bowls and spoons that can be sterilised
- Hand blender. The really cheap, simple ones are by far the best, as you will be able to control how much or little you purée the food. This really helps as your baby gets older and you want to purée the food slightly but still leave it a bit lumpy
- Six ice cube trays. The rubber ones that the cubes can easily be pushed out of are the most helpful. Plastic ones are fine if you can't get hold of the others though; it is very easy to use a clean knife to ease the cubes out of the trays
- Tie-handle freezer bags

- Steamer or three-tier saucepan steaming pans
- Bibs. Plastic-backed ones are the best once you start weaning, as food tends to stain the bib and go through on to a baby's clothes if you buy the material ones

You can prepare a batch of a few different fruits and vegetables a few weeks before your baby is ready for weaning and have them already stored as frozen cubes in your freezer. You will then be able to simply take one cube out of the freezer the night before and place in a bowl in the fridge to defrost overnight. You can then heat it up the following day.

The first foods that I would recommend buying are:

- Carrots
- Apples
- Sweet potato
- Pears
- Broccoli
- Cauliflower
- Courgettes
- Tomatoes

Buy a couple of bags of each item. They will need to be cut, peeled and cooked before you can purée them. You can either boil the fruit or vegetables (each one separately) in a pan of water or steam them. Steaming to soften them is the best way to ensure that all of the nutrients and goodness is not lost – something that can happen when they are boiled.

Directions
- Steam or boil one lot of fruit or vegetables at a time.
- Once soft, place in a jug or bowl and use your hand blender to purée. Ensure that there are absolutely no lumps and that the purée is completely smooth.

- Spoon into the ice cube tray(s) until you have no purée left in your bowl.
- Place the trays in a freezer overnight.
- The following day, push out each frozen cube of purée and place into your labelled freezer bag. Ensure you write the date on the bag, as well as details of the contents.
- Tie the handles once finished and place back into your freezer. Plain fruit and vegetables can be stored as cubes in the freezer for up to six months.

Tip

Always test the purée with a clean spoon before offering it to your baby, to ensure it will not burn her.

If you follow the above instructions for a variety of fruit and vegetables, you will end up with a whole variety in your freezer, which you can use when needed. It can then be heated by placing in a small saucepan and stirring until hot, or heated in a microwave. Heat until piping hot and stir thoroughly to prevent any hot spots. Leave to cool to the right temperature.

Tip

It is recommended that you only introduce a new fruit or vegetable to your baby every two to three days. This is so that you will be able to pinpoint any foods that may cause an allergic reaction to your baby. This is another good reason for giving your baby home-cooked purées in the early stages of weaning in particular. You will then know exactly what she has eaten. In the case of jars or packets of food, they usually have a few different ingredients, so it is harder to pinpoint exactly what may have caused any reaction right away.

Initially you should only offer your baby a single fruit or vegetable to try. The watery ones, like apple, pear, tomato and courgette, can be mixed with a little baby rice to thicken them up a bit. Later on you will be able to mix two or three cubes of different vegetables together to make her meals a little more tasty and varied.

Foods to definitely avoid completely in the first 12 months

- **Honey**. *Some honey can contain a type of bacteria which produces toxins in your baby's intestines and causes a very serious illness called infant botulism.*
- **Nuts**. *This is mainly due to the risk of choking, but also due to the risk of allergies. If there is a family history then it would be best to avoid nuts altogether until your baby is at least two to three years old.*
- **Salt**. *Don't add this to your baby's food, and be careful to avoid foods that may contain a lot of salt. Your baby's kidneys will not be developed enough to cope with this substance.*
- **Sugar**. *This can lead to tooth decay or, worst-case scenario, your baby's top teeth could come through black. I saw this happen to a friend's baby when I was a teenager. He was regularly allowed to suck on sugar cubes as he enjoyed them and his mother didn't see any harm in it. I think she regretted allowing him to do it though when his four top teeth came through as black stumps and stayed that way until they fell out at six years old, when his new teeth came through.*

  Giving juice to your baby in a bottle can also cause this to happen too. They will be sucking the juice directly on to their gums, which is why it is one of my pet hates to see a baby drinking juice out of a bottle. If you want to give her juice rather than water, then offer it to her in a cup or beaker.
- **Shark, swordfish, king mackerel, marlin or tilefish**. *This is because they all contain high levels of mercury, which can harm a*

young child's developing nervous system. **Shellfish** also runs the risk of giving your baby food poisoning.

- **High-fibre, low-fat or low-calorie foods**. Having too much fibre can stop your baby absorbing enough iron and calcium, and babies do not need 'diet foods'.
- **Cow's milk** to drink should not be given until your baby is over one year. It can still be used in foods from the age of six months, when making up recipes that require its use, e.g., cheese sauces.

Below is a guideline that can be used to help you get started on weaning. All foods and spoons that the baby is fed from should be sterilised for the first few weeks. After this, putting them in a dishwasher or washing them thoroughly with hot, soapy water will be sufficient. You can then just run them under boiling water from the kettle immediately before use to kill off any major germs. If you would prefer to keep sterilising them though, that is fine too.

When you offer your baby food from a spoon it's important you allow her to get used to the new experience gradually. If you just push the food straight into her mouth she is likely to gag, and possibly choke. During the first few weeks of weaning you need to almost tease your baby with the spoon. Put the spoon up to her lips and let her taste this new thing you are offering her. I'm sure you will get a variety of strange faces pulled at you. This is normal and doesn't mean she has taken an immediate dislike to the new taste. Like every new experience, she just needs time to practise at it and get used to it. Allow her to suck the food off the spoon. As she takes it into her mouth tilt the spoon upwards. This will help the food come off the spoon and into her mouth, and it creates slightly less mess around her mouth.

Try just a few spoonfuls the first few times you introduce a new taste. It's a good idea to stop before she gets completely fed up and refuses any more. This will go a long way to giving her good food associations and not learning that she needs to cry when she's had enough. I've always made a point of saying 'last one' and then 'all gone' to any baby I feed. It's good to teach them this from a young age, and they pick it up and understand what you mean pretty quickly. This is helpful for when you are feeding them something savoury in a few months, but they have learned that pudding comes next. The cues above will give them an indication and encouragement to keep going.

Tip

Some babies like to hold their own spoon as you are feeding them, or even a small toy of some kind. It gives them something to wave around and distracts them as you are feeding them. You may want to save this distraction tip for halfway through their meal or when their attention to eat begins to wane. In giving them a spoon or toy you can usually manage to get a few extra spoonfuls of purée into them.

A two-week weaning guide

Days 1–3
Time: 11 a.m. feed
Food: Baby rice – 1 tsp mixed with breast milk or formula until it reaches a very smooth consistency
Direction: Give three-quarters of her usual formula feed first, or one full breast. Wind as usual, then offer solids. Give any remaining milk in the bottle, or the second breast after solids

Days 4–6
Time: 11 a.m. feed
Food: 1 cube pear purée
Directions: As above

Time: 6 p.m.
Food: Baby rice
Directions: Give as above. Increase from 1 tsp in quantity each day.
Be guided by your baby as to what is enough

Days 7–9
Time: 11 a.m. feed
Food: Sweet potato
Directions: Keep giving three-quarters of milk feed before solids,
then allow her to finish the remaining milk

Time: 6 p.m. feed
Food: 1 cube of pear purée mixed with baby rice
Directions: As above

Days 10–12
Time: 11 a.m. feed
Food: 1 cube of carrot purée
Directions: As above

Time: 6 p.m. feed
Food: 1–2 cubes of pear purée mixed with baby rice
Directions: As above, but be guided by your baby as to what is the
correct amount

Days 13–15
Time: 11 a.m. feed
Food: Alternate carrot and sweet potato, or mix together
Directions: As above. Be guided by your baby as to the amounts

Time: 6 p.m. feed
Food: Apple purée mixed with baby rice
Directions: As above

Continue to introduce a new vegetable or fruit every two to three days from the freezer stock list. At this stage it's advisable to always give the vegetable at the morning feed and the fruit at the bedtime feed.

Tip

Bananas can be mashed or puréed but any purée needs to be used immediately. You cannot freeze banana purée.

If your baby has experienced a particular fruit or vegetable and not shown an adverse reaction to it, then you can begin mixing various ones together to create new tastes for her. For example:

- Carrot and broccoli
- Sweet potato and cauliflower
- Apple and pear

Once she has had a large variety of fruits and vegetables you can begin to introduce protein and dairy into her diet as soon as she's over 6 months old. These can be mixed with the vegetables that your baby already enjoys.

Making a chicken casserole is usually a good way to introduce your baby to her first tastes of protein. You can also do casseroles made with lamb and beef. I had a few recipes that were very easy to make in large quantities and still freeze them into cubes once puréed. I found this easier to do than freezing separate portions of each recipe in pots or bowls, which I felt would take up more space. Some people prefer this method though – whatever works best for each individual parent is fine.

Annabel Karmel has a very good cookbook for babies with very simple instructions on how to make a variety of recipes. I picked some favourites from her book that were a big hit with all three of my children, and then also made some traditional meals of my own. I then alternated different meals on different days over the course of a week.

Meal examples include:

- Casseroles: chicken, lamb, beef and vegetable
- Shepherd's pie
- Lasagne
- Mild chilli with rice
- Cod in a cheesy white sauce
- Salmon in chive sauce (Annabel Karmel – AK)
- Sausage casserole
- Lovely lentils (AK)
- Chicken in tomato sauce (AK)
- Cheesy spinach pasta (AK)
- Pasta with courgettes and tomato (AK)
- Cauliflower and broccoli cheese – I also added bits of ham chopped up and carrots as my children got older to make this meal more interesting and lumpier

Once you introduce protein and dairy, it is very easy to just cook large batches of recipes like the ones listed above, and purée or freeze them as cubes. You will then have a freezer bag of each meal as cubes. The correct quantity can then be taken out the night before to defrost in the fridge overnight, for the following day's meal. As your baby gets older her appetite will increase, so you will need to be guided by her as to how many cubes are enough for each meal. Every baby's appetite is different, even between siblings or twins. As already mentioned, cow's milk can be used in foods given to your baby but she cannot have it to drink in a cup or bottle until she is over 12 months.

You can also begin to introduce your baby to two courses at each meal, e.g., a vegetable- or protein-based meal, and then a sweet fruit or pudding type of dessert afterwards.

The early-morning poo

In my experience, if a baby has a protein-based meal that includes meat at teatime, it can cause them to wake before 7 a.m. with an early-morning poo! I discovered this with my first child, and as soon as I stopped giving him a meat-based meal at teatime the problem was solved. I have always advised the mothers I work with to do this too. Some have forgotten once I leave and they get to the weaning stage, and then contact me to say, 'She's waking with a dirty nappy at 5:30 some mornings, and is then difficult to resettle once I change her – what do I do?' As soon as I remind them about the no-meat rule at teatime, they remember, and once it is cut out again the problem resolves itself! By only giving a meat-based meal at lunchtime, the baby has time to produce a soiled nappy long before bedtime.

Desserts or puddings

There are various foods that can be given as puddings or dessert:

- *Yoghurt*
- *Fruit purée*
- *Banana*
- *Custard*
- *Rice pudding*
- *Jelly*

You can also introduce water in a cup or beaker to offer her with her two meals. There are various cups and beakers available to buy. I have found the free-flow cups are the best by far, as your baby won't have to work really hard on this type of cup to get the water to come out. It will spill into her mouth as soon as she, or you, tip it up with the spout in her mouth. It's also better to buy one with handles to encourage and teach her how to hold the cup herself from a young age.

The cup that I bought for all three of my children, and that I always recommend to friends and clients, is the 'first cup' by Tommee Tippee. It's very cheap, priced at £1.99, and is lightweight, easy to drink from and can also be used from baby right through to toddlerhood. You can just remove the lid as she gets older to teach her how to drink like a big girl! These cups can be bought in three different colours – blue, green and pink – and are available at all major supermarkets, or directly from the Tommee Tippee website.

Taking milk from a cup rather than a bottle

Later on when you decide to wean your baby off the bottle altogether and drink milk from a cup or beaker, I would advise buying a separate and altogether different type of beaker. Once you have her established at drinking a regular amount of water from the cup every day, then it is a bad idea to confuse her by putting milk in the same cup! She will associate her cup with water and the bottle or breast with milk, and you may put her off the water cup you have established by beginning to put milk into it.

Choose a similar free-flow type of cup, but ensure it looks different. Most babies and toddlers resist the idea of giving up their bottle altogether and having to get used to the idea of having milk from a cup instead. They generally reduce the amount of milk they will drink dramatically when you change to a beaker/cup of milk instead of their usual bottle. This is normal and eventually most will begin to drink milk again, but it usually takes a period of weeks rather than days. Due to the fact that it does take a couple of weeks for your child to get used to the idea, and during this time she is likely to have a lower milk intake, I would give two pieces of advice:

- That you wait until she is over one year. The guidelines on the recommended minimum milk intake drops from 20fl oz

(600ml) a day for a baby under one year, to 10–12fl oz (300–360ml) for babies over 12 months (inclusive of milk used in foods as well as milk drank). If your baby reduces her milk intake too quickly because you have changed her over to a cup, it will be more difficult for you to make up the difference in foods she eats if she is under one year, and needing a minimum of 20fl oz (600ml) per day. It's much easier if you only need to ensure that she gets 11fl oz (330ml) per day!

- Generally by 12 months most babies will only be on two milk feeds per day: once first thing in the morning when she wakes and one last thing at night around 6:30 p.m., before she goes to bed.

Change the morning bottle- or breastfeed to a cup first, and make sure she is well established and drinking a regular amount from the cup in the morning before you try to change the bedtime milk feed. The risk of changing her bedtime milk to a cup too soon may mean she could potentially wake hungry in the night if she decreases her milk intake in response to you introducing a cup. You can change the bedtime milk to a cup in a more gradual way, to ensure she is still taking an adequate amount every night. Offer her a cup of milk first, and then, if you feel that she hasn't taken an adequate amount of milk to enable her to sleep all night, you can always offer her a top-up from the breast or bottle before she goes to bed. As time goes by she will naturally increase the amount of milk she takes from the cup as she gets used to it, and you will feel less inclined to offer her a top-up, until she is weaned off the breast or bottle completely.

Jars/pre-prepared packet food

Although I would recommend providing your baby with home-prepared food most of the time, it is a good idea to also get her used to the taste of a jar of food bought from the supermarket. This is so that you know she will eat from them if you ever need to give her one to eat on a day out or on holiday, for example. It is very easy from a parent's point of view to take a bowl of home-cooked food out with you, but you may struggle at times to find somewhere to heat it up. Some shops or places of interest will refuse to heat up your home-cooked purées for fear of 'contaminating' their microwave! They state that it is due to health and safety hygiene laws in their workplace. They will, however, allow you to heat up jarred food if you show them that it is sealed before you open it.

I've always offered my babies a supermarket-bought organic jar once a week, or once a fortnight, just to get them used to the taste. Despite there being a variety of meals offered from various baby food companies, they all seem to taste very similar, and, in my opinion, not too tasty or appetising at all. I have often finished the last few spoonfuls of my baby's home-cooked meals if she had finished and didn't want any more, however I can't say the same for the pre-prepared jars or packet meals!

The exceptions are the fruit purée pots or squeezy pouches. These can be bought as single fruits – just apple or just pears etc. – or with a few fruits mixed together. They are all very tasty to eat and you can really tell the differences in the fruits used in terms of flavour. They can also be bought containing some of the more exotic fruits too like pineapple, watermelon, mango, black- or redcurrants, etc. It is great for your baby to experience these tastes too, especially as they are probably fruits that you may not necessarily think to cook and purée at home.

Introducing lumps and finger foods

First finger foods like toast, rusks, rice cakes, and banana can be offered to your baby from around seven months of age. The various foods you offer her need to be big enough for her to pick up and hold, and should not have any bones, pips or stones in. You can also offer various steamed vegetables.

Please note

Remember never to leave your baby alone while she is feeding herself – it is amazing how quickly babies can choke!

Toast is a great first finger food to give your baby to try. You will find she will probably just suck it until it goes very soggy. It's important that you then take this soggy bit away and give her a fresh piece, as she's more likely to gag and choke on the leftover soggy bits.

If your baby does start gagging and choking like she has a piece of toast or any other finger food stuck in her throat, then you need to stay calm and act quickly.

Generally a good hard pat on the back as she is sitting upright will be enough to dislodge anything that has got stuck in her throat. Sometimes it can take three or four pats for it to work. Understandably, every parent's natural reaction is to panic the first time they see this happen to their baby. However, your baby is more likely to panic too if she sees you losing control, which will add to the problem. Try to stay calm on the outside, even though your heart will be racing. It is very common for babies to gag and choke every now and then as you introduce her to lumps and finger foods. Talk to her to calm her as you are patting her back to calm her down. Quite often a baby will be a little bit sick when the piece of food is dislodged, as the gag reflex helps her to bring up whatever she has just eaten. Usually it is just a small amount, but occasionally it can be the entire meal, which is very frustrating. They also tend to cry afterwards too as the whole thing is a bit scary! Again, reassure her with your voice and try to distract her with something to calm her down.

Generally babies are able to eat various finger foods quite happily before they are ready to eat lumpier food from a spoon. It really varies from baby to baby, even among twins, as to when they are ready to take food that hasn't been completely puréed from a spoon. Even though she may seem to cope perfectly well with eating and swallowing lots of different textured food, you may offer her to hold and eat with her hands, which is a different experience to taking it off a spoon.

The presence of teeth also doesn't seem to make a difference to when your baby will accept lumpier foods from a spoon. A baby aged eight months with no teeth may happily begin taking lumpier meals, when equally a baby aged 12 months with five teeth may still spit out any kind of lumpy food you give her and only accept completely puréed food!

CASE STUDY: My three and lumpy food

My three children, despite being siblings, were all completely different as to when they accepted lumpier food:

Number 1: Got his first tooth at 11 months. Was eating various finger foods from seven months and lumpier food from a spoon from eight or nine months.

Number 2: First tooth at 13 and a half months. Refused any lumpy food off a spoon until he was well over a year old. If I tried to feed him any kind of purée that had some lumps mixed in, he would just spit the mouthful of food straight back out again every time! He was eating a range of various finger foods from around seven or eight months though, so I knew he could cope with chewing, he just wasn't ready for lumps from a spoon. I just kept going back to the puréed food and then trying him again on a lumpier meal a couple of weeks later again. He began accepting them more and more from around 14 months onwards.

Number 3: First tooth at 13 months. Eating various finger foods from seven months and happy to eat lumpy food from a spoon from eight or nine months too.

It is actually the molars that do any major chewing for babies, children and adults. Obviously, these don't generally come through for most babies until they are over 12 months of age anyway, which is why you need to be careful with what foods you offer your baby. Her gums will be very hard even without the teeth having cut, which is how she copes with the finger foods and lumps that you do offer to her.

Whenever I made foods slightly lumpier than the usual purée, I would try a small spoonful myself, and try to swallow it without chewing it at all and using my own teeth. If I found I was unable to do this, then I knew it was unlikely my baby would be able to. It is always worth trying your particular baby with a small spoonful and gauging her reaction – she may surprise you and eat it happily!

My school of thinking has always been that babies that do not have any development issues are generally eating a range of lumpy food from a spoon by the age of two, regardless of the age that they began to do it. I always tell parents not to worry if their baby is refusing lumps off a spoon, as long as she is happily eating and coping with various finger foods. They all get to the same stage eventually – some just get there a little bit quicker than others. As always, be guided by your baby on this and, with the usual patience and perseverance, she will get there in the end.

The most crucial thing to remember is, like bottle- or breast-feeding, it is important not to make your baby's meal times a stressful or pressured time. There will be days when she eats a large amount of solids and other days where she is only happy to take a small amount. This is normal and nothing to get stressed about. If you add up the total amount of solids she eats over an entire week and average it out, then you will most likely find that she has taken in enough food to sustain herself.

Illnesses and viruses will have an impact on your baby's appetite, as is the case when we as adults get ill. In my experience it tends to be the solids that babies go off when they are feeling ill or under the weather, but they still seem to enjoy the comfort of their milk feed. It's important that you don't try to force her or make her feel pressured to eat. Offer her the solids as you normally would, but try not to worry if she refuses to eat a lot or even anything at all over a few days when suffering from a virus. As long as she's drinking enough fluids between her milk intake and any boiled water you offer her too, then her appetite is likely to pick up when she is feeling better again. Babies tend to eat like a horse the week after they have been ill, as their way of trying to make up for the recent lower intake of food!

In my opinion, one thing I think it is helpful to teach your baby about is when the meal is finished and what happens next. To teach this I always say 'last one' to every baby I feed solids to as I am giving the final spoonful. I then make a point of showing the baby the empty bowl and saying 'all gone!' If you do this from the early stages of weaning, then you will find that your baby will very quickly learn what these words mean. Once you start to give two courses – savoury and then dessert – she will also begin to understand that she gets something sweeter after her main meal.

At times you may find that your baby may be struggling to eat the regular amount of food that she usually eats. To still manage to do the 'last one, all gone' saying you have to be a bit sneaky in this situation. To follow this through, you can scoop some of the food from the bowl into the bin, leaving just a couple of spoonfuls left. (Make sure you do this without her seeing you put the excess food in the bin though – it's amazing how clever babies are, and can figure out what you are up to!) You can then offer her the final spoonfuls and repeat the usual 'last one' and 'all gone', as you show her the empty bowl.

In her eyes you are in control of the meal and how much she is eating, rather than her. It sounds ridiculous, but just sticking to a simple rule like this encourages her to finish her meals as she's got some idea of when the end is near. This is particularly important with her main meal, before you offer her the dessert or sweet pudding.

Babies learn very quickly that their sweet part of the meal comes after the savoury. Some will protest about eating the savoury part because they know the dessert is on its way. As long as you can get a few spoonfuls of the savoury meal into her and do the 'last one, all gone' phrases, and show her the empty bowl, she will learn that she has to finish her main meal before the treat comes from a very early age. If she does refuse the savoury part of the meal completely, then it's a bad idea to offer her something sweet in return. Wait until the next time she is due to be offered solids and try her again with savoury first and then dessert if she happily eats some savoury.

It is very easy for a baby to slip into bad eating habits, but it is much harder for them to be broken! Instilling good eating habits from a very early age encourages your baby to continue with them as they get older. Only you can teach that, and following the simple rule above will go a long way to getting there.

The 'last one, all gone,' saying can also be used in many other situations too as your baby gets older. Washing her hair by pouring a cup of water over her head, last go on a swing in the park, are just a couple of examples. Babies and children love to have cues and warnings that something is going to stop, and because she has learnt to recognise what this saying means from an early age it is very helpful, and can prevent a major tantrum at times!

Establishing the three main meals

According to government guidelines a baby under one year should have a minimum intake of 20fl oz (600ml) of breast milk or infant formula milk per day to aid development and help them stay healthy.

When you begin weaning and eventually start to introduce dairy into her diet, then you can include the milk used in the foods you give her to help make up this daily intake. White/cheese sauces, rice pudding and custard can all be given an estimated value in millilitres or ounces, depending on portion sizes, and added to the total daily amount of milk intake, on top of what she takes from the breast or bottle.

As an example the value that I gave foods that I offered my babies were as follows:

1 small yoghurt = 1fl oz (30ml)
1 portion of white/cheese sauce = 1–2fl oz (30–60ml)
1 portion of custard made with milk = 1–2fl oz (30–60ml)
1 portion of rice pudding = 1fl oz (30ml)

The above was purely my own guesswork – this is not supported or copied by any healthcare guide – and is just to give you a guide of how you can incorporate milk values in food into your baby's daily intake.

By five to six months when you begin weaning, your baby will most likely have already dropped her 3/4 a.m. night feed, particularly if you have been following the feed and sleep times in this book since birth. If she is still having her night feed then please see advice on how to drop the night feed on page 137 of the feeding section.

She should now be on four to five breast- or bottle-feeds per day, at roughly the following times:

- 7/7:45 a.m.
- 11 a.m.
- 2:30 p.m.
- 6/6:15 p.m.
- 10:30 p.m. (Some babies may have dropped this before weaning – see advice in feeding section.)

As discussed, the plan would be to introduce solids at the 11 a.m. and 6 p.m. feeds. Initially you should continue to give your baby most of her milk intake before the solids offered at both of these feeds. After a number of weeks you should have been able to offer your baby a wide variety of fruit and vegetables. You will then reach the stage where you are ready to introduce protein and dairy into her diet. Ideas of different meals to offer containing these food groups have already been discussed. It is also very important that you ensure your baby gets enough foods containing iron after the age of six months as the iron stores that a full-term, healthy baby was born with can sometimes begin to drop. This is more likely if your baby has been exclusively formula fed, without any breast milk. Once you wean your baby, it is very easy to ensure she gets enough iron intake by giving her the correct foods containing plenty of iron.

Foods that are high in iron
- *Meat and poultry*
- *Sweet potato*
- *Spinach*
- *Dried beans (e.g., kidney beans, lentils)*

The current research indicates that a baby's iron stores should last between six and twelve months, depending upon the baby, if she has been completely breastfed.

Lunch

When you begin to introduce protein and dairy into your baby's diet at this meal you can then begin to reduce and drop the milk feed that she also has – whether it is from the breast or bottle. Giving milk to drink at the same time as certain foods that contain iron can affect how well the iron is absorbed into a baby's body, so it's important to drop this milk feed as soon as you can.

Some mothers choose to move this milk feed back to 10:15/ 10:30 a.m. and then give the solids slightly later at 11:15 a.m. if their baby is not a big milk drinker and they are struggling to get the minimum daily milk intake into them. If however your baby is taking the required amount of milk on a daily basis then it's best to drop this milk feed altogether. Giving too much milk may put a baby off solids, as she won't have an appetite for them. Solids are very important though after the age of six months to ensure your baby replenishes any iron stores already used up by this age!

Reduce and drop the milk feed using the following process:

- Reduce the amount that you put into her bottle by 1fl oz (30ml) every three days. If you are breastfeeding at this time then allow her five minutes less over the entire feed every three days.
- Continue to give her milk feed first, before any solids.
- Introduce a cup of cool boiled water with her protein-based meal. She can be offered and encouraged to have sips from it in between spoonfuls of her food. Baby juice is unnecessary, as all babies will drink water if you persevere with it and continue to offer it every day. It is bound to take her a period of weeks rather than days to start to drink a regular amount at meal times. This will be the case whether you give her cool boiled water, or well-diluted juice, and in the long run it is better to get her used to, and liking, the taste of water from a very young age!
- Once you have the milk feed down to 2fl oz (60ml) or five minutes on the breast for three days in a row, then you can drop the milk feed completely.
- As soon as you stop the milk at this time then you can introduce pudding/dessert to your baby after her protein-based meal. Various suggestions for dessert have already been mentioned.
- The solids given at 11 a.m. can be gradually pushed to a later time closer to a usual family lunchtime of 12 p.m., as your baby gets older. Breakfast should be introduced before this can happen. It is also important that she is not too tired when you try to feed her at a later time (particularly if she has already dropped her morning nap). You will find that she is unlikely to eat very well if she is too tired, which in turn could affect how well she sleeps during her lunchtime nap.

Breakfast

This meal should only be introduced when your baby begins to show signs of finding it increasingly harder to wait from her 7/7:45 a.m. milk feed to the 11 a.m. milk and solids feed. You will probably notice that from 10 a.m. onwards she may begin to get grumpy and less happy to play during this time, where previously she would have waited patiently. If you introduce a small amount of cereal around 8 a.m. after her morning bottle- or breastfeed she should then go back to being her previous happy self between 10 and 11 a.m., leading up to the lunchtime solids.

Please note

It is very important that you don't introduce breakfast before your baby starts to show the hunger signs that she is ready. If you begin to give her breakfast too soon, then you run the risk that the solids she takes then will put her off her 11 a.m. feed. This will in turn affect her lunchtime nap if she wakes hungry because she hasn't fed well at 11 a.m. It's very easy for simple changes, made too soon, to have a profound affect on every part of her day.

As usual, be guided by your baby and wait until she is ready, rather than you giving her the extra meal because you feel pressured by the fact that friends' babies are having it, and you feel it is the next step your baby should also be taking. Don't worry – she will get there in her own time, and let you know for sure when she needs anything extra.

Tea

There will come a time when, despite having her 2:30 p.m. milk feed from the breast or bottle as normal, you notice that your baby begins to get grumpy and show signs of hunger from 4:15 p.m. onwards. Rather than reintroducing her 5 p.m. milk top-up feed, now is the time to bring her solids forward from the current time of 6 p.m. with her milk feed, to between 4:30 and 5 p.m. Ideally I would suggest offering it to her at 4:30 p.m. initially, as a test to make sure she is still happy to take her normal amount of milk after 6 p.m.

- You can offer a vegetable- or pasta-based meal at this time followed by dessert. (See earlier suggestions on page 252.)
- Offer her a drink of cool boiled water in a cup with her meal.
- The feed can eventually be brought forward to 5 p.m., which most people feel is a more normal time for tea. Make sure that she continues to take a good amount of milk before bed and is not too full from having the solids at 5 p.m. You can always move it back to 4:30 p.m. if it does seem to have an impact on her milk feed, and then try pushing it towards 5 p.m. again a month or two later.
- Depending on how much sleep she has had in the afternoon, you may be able to push her current 6/6:15 p.m. milk time to a slightly later feed time of 6:30/6:45 p.m. This would depend how tired she is though, as you don't want to run the risk of her only taking a small feed because she's too tired to persevere in having her usual full breast- or bottle-feed.

By 12 months the majority of babies are usually on the three main meals – breakfast, lunch and tea – and two milk feeds per day: one first thing in the morning when they wake and one last thing in the evening, before bed.

7

Common problems and illnesses for Mum and Baby

There are a number of common problems and illnesses that many new parents encounter in the first year and I thought it would be helpful to list some of them here and what you can do.

Teething
Pain and crying are just one symptom of teething. There are various other signs that your baby could be teething:

- Dribbling (The mouth produces more saliva when a baby teethes. It's too much for them to swallow continuously so they dribble it out)
- Chewing hands or fists (Helps ease the painful gums)
- One or both cheeks may be red and hot to touch (Usually on the side of the mouth which is causing the pain)
- Looser poos than normal (The extra saliva produced, which is swallowed, upsets a baby's tummy slightly, and causes her to produce more acidic poos)
- Red, sore bottom (Due to the acidic poos)
- Pulling at her ears (A sign of pain on one side of the mouth)
- Decreased appetite – refusing to drink her milk or eat solids (Mouth may be too sore)

- Generally whingy or unhappy (If teeth are just having a rumble and causing a small amount of pain)
- Unexplained bouts of screaming hysterically which nothing you do seems to relieve (Very bad teething pain)
- Not sleeping well. Whinging or moaning in her sleep or waking up screaming (Due to pain)

If your baby is showing at least three of the above signs then you can say with a fair amount of certainty that it is likely to be teething pain that is the problem. Many parents will notice a few more unusual signs every time their baby is about to cut a tooth – e.g., they always develop a cold – but I have tried to stick to the more common signs above that are normal in the majority of babies.

> **Please note**
>
> *If she seems in pain but doesn't show any of the other symptoms above, then I would recommend that you talk to your GP for more advice.*

A baby who is teething will not self-soothe or calm herself down until the pain has stopped. If it happens during the night she will wake repeatedly, crying. She may settle initially with a cuddle if it is just mild teething pain, but will likely be unsettled and wake on and off all night. With more severe pain she will be almost hysterical, and crying even when comforted. Most adults will have experienced toothache or pain when wisdom teeth are having a 'rumble' for a few days and trying to push through the gums. It can even put you off eating because your mouth is so sore – but at least we understand what is going on and can self-medicate accordingly. A baby has no idea what is happening and the only way to let her parent know is to cry.

Unfortunately, teething is one of those things that goes on for months, sometimes without any results. Symptoms can begin from the age of eight to ten weeks, although some babies have been known to be born with teeth or get a couple very early on! For the majority, teeth can take a very long time to appear. They rumble in the gums, gradually pushing their way up before 'erupting' (aptly named by dentists) and 'cutting' through the gum so that you can finally feel the sharp tip and see it. It's normal for a baby to suffer with teething pain for two to three days, and show the various signs above, and then be fine again for a few weeks.

Babies vary at the age and order in which teeth erupt in their mouth. Here is a diagram to give you a rough idea of when to expect things.

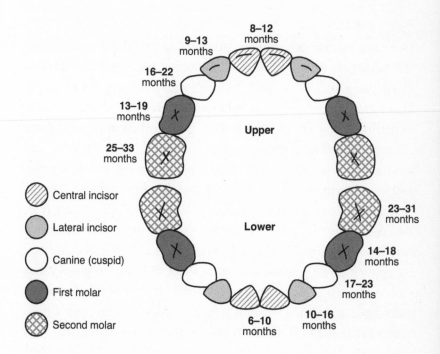

However, please do not panic if your baby doesn't fit in with 'the norms' above. None of my three children have conformed to this diagram, and the same goes for many other babies. It is just a rough guide.

My first son got a top tooth, then a bottom side tooth, then a top side and then a bottom front, all within the space of four weeks, between the ages of 11 and 12 months.

My second son was different again – he was completely gummy until almost 14 months. I thought he would never get teeth!

My daughter got her bottom two incisors then the top four incisors and then her four molars. We were still waiting for her lateral incisors at 18 months!

All teeth arrive eventually in their own order, in their own time. It feels like a long haul as you and she are dealing with all the pain and symptoms, but you get there in the end!

Treatment

There are various gels, liquids, powders and teething products on the market, as well as necklaces containing particular ingredients, all claiming to be the best to help with teething pain. In my experience, after trying a number of different products with my own three children and the babies I've worked with, and from chatting to other mums, I have found the most helpful and soothing product to be a teething liquid called Anbesol. It's also sold in gel form too, but I've found that, like other gels, it slips off the gums and around the mouth as you are attempting to apply it. This means that you don't really get enough of it on to the gums to relieve the pain. The liquid is much more effective because you can apply it directly along your baby's top and bottom gums using a clean fingertip. It contains an antiseptic ingredient as well as an anaesthetic so it brings instant relief. In using this product I have noticed that it has worked to relieve the pain, whereas if I had been using something else that wasn't as effective, I would have had to resort to giving infant paracetamol or Nurofen to relieve the pain. Although it is perfectly safe to use products like baby Calpol and Nurofen for pain once your baby is over 8–12 weeks, they will lose the benefits they bring in relieving pain if used too frequently, just like any medicine does.

The Anbesol liquid is so good but if you find that it isn't working on relieving the pain and your baby continues to be distressed, then Calpol or Nurofen is your final option. I personally found Calpol good for relieving mild temperatures and mild teething pain. However, when the pain was very severe, only Nurofen would work on my babies. It takes 20 minutes to get to work and after that they are pain-free and a much happier baby.

Once you have eliminated her pain, then you can attempt to get her to calm down and settle back to sleep (if at night).

Coughs and colds

In my experience the majority of babies tend to develop their first little cold by the age of six to eight weeks, whether they are born in the summer or the winter. If your baby is your second or third child though, and already has older siblings, then it is more likely that she will develop a cold earlier with the germs being brought home from school or nursery by her siblings.

You may notice she sounds very snuffly and bunged up and may even be snorting a lot and sound like a little piggy, as she tries to breathe through her blocked nostrils. Being so bunged up in her nose may also make it more difficult for her to feed. Usually when she drinks and swallows she would be breathing through her nose. If she has a cold this will be more difficult to do and she will get tired a lot quicker as she feeds, from the extra effort she has to put in. She may also cough and splutter more or even vomit after a feed, as she tries to coordinate the sucking, swallowing and breathing all at the same time.

Treatment

The recommended treatment by doctors and pharmacists to begin with is to use saline nasal drops. This is basically sterile water in a bottle and can be squirted up her nose before a feed. The water irritates her bunged-up nose and causes her to sneeze almost immediately. This is exactly what you need to happen to help unblock her nose. Babies cannot blow their noses so this helps to relieve the problem. Squirting the nasal drops up each nostril before a feed and making her sneeze will help ease her stuffiness and hopefully enable her to feed easier.

Other things to try when she is sleeping:

- Prop the Moses basket/cot up at the head end by placing books etc. under the feet. This puts her sleeping position at more of a slant to help her breathe better.
- You can also put a towel/blanket under her mattress if you want to. This will also slant her sleeping position to help her breathe easier.
- If you aren't already lying her on her side to sleep as suggested and explained in Chapter 5, then you may want to consider it now, even if it is only while she has a cold. Lying on her back will make it much harder for her to breathe. I'm sure as an adult you can relate to having had a heavy cold in the past and how much more difficult it is to breathe on your back. Lying her on her side will help her to breathe easier and sleep better.

If she develops a cough with her cold then always get it checked by a doctor as some cold viruses can lead to chest infections or croup (see below and page 275).

Chest infections

Most chest infections are caused by a virus, which is spread from one person to another by coughing or sneezing. Your baby may have had a cold for a while that develops into a cough. Chest infections attack the airways in the lungs so they become inflamed and filled with mucus. An infection can clog up a baby's air passages more easily than older children or adults because they are much smaller. It can then be more difficult for her to breathe and can make her wheezy or feverish with a cough.

Bronchiolitis is one of the most common chest infections in babies and is caused by a virus called respiratory syncytial virus (RSV), which is most likely to strike during the winter months between October and March. It affects about one in three babies in their first year. Premature babies, whose immune systems are less able to fight off infections, are particularly susceptible to RSV, especially if they are born in the winter during the first few months after birth.

First symptoms caused by the virus are usually mild:

- Runny or stuffy nose
- Dry cough
- Mild fever of between 37.5 and 38°C (99.5 and 100.4°F)
- Loss of appetite

After two to three days, symptoms may peak:

- Cough may be more persistent
- Breathing may become faster and sound shallow and laboured
- Heartbeat may be much faster
- There may be trouble feeding or she may refuse feeds

Treatment

Most cases of bronchiolitis get better on their own within a week or two. Doctors don't tend to prescribe antibiotics, as they are only effective in treating bacterial infections, rather than viral ones.

Advised treatments to relieve above symptoms are:

- Infant paracetamol or ibuprofen (minimum age 12 weeks). This will help reduce any high temperature and relieve a sore throat, encouraging her to feed more easily.
- Short frequent feeds to prevent her becoming dehydrated if she is taking less milk at her usual feed times. Top-ups in between may be necessary.
- Saline nasal drops to relieve a stuffy nose – use before feeds to help unblock her nostrils. Sit her as upright as possible during feeds.

- Breathing in steam can help loosen mucus blocking your baby's airways and relieve her cough. Sit in the bathroom with your baby for a few minutes while the shower or hot taps are running. The steam that is created and circulated around the room will help her breathe more easily. Remember to change her clothes after doing this though, as they may be damp from the steam.

If you are worried at any point that your baby doesn't seem to be improving then see your doctor as soon as possible. Some babies need to be prescribed an inhaler if their breathing continues to be laboured and wheezy to help them get over the bronchiolitis. This doesn't necessarily mean the inhaler will be a long-term thing and that your baby has asthma.

Both my second son and daughter suffered from chest infections as babies. At 17 months my daughter ended up on three different inhalers per day during a particularly bad case of bronchiolitis until she got over it a week later. Amazingly she was still very chirpy, running around, smiling and laughing – despite the fact that her breathing made her sound like a chain smoker!

Any illness caused by a virus like RSV is very contagious. Viruses are passed on by touching, so they spread very quickly in places like nurseries, offices and even homes. They can live on hands and surfaces for up to six hours, so practising good hygiene can help prevent your baby catching them. Wash your hands with warm water and soap if you have been outside of the home before holding your baby, and encourage visitors to do the same.

There are so many different viruses that it is impossible to shield your baby from them all forever. Staying in the house and locking yourself away will only delay the inevitable. Eventually you will have to take your baby out, and she will end up with a cough, cold or some other viral infection. This is a perfectly normal part of developing and growing up. It's important that she builds up immunity to viruses. The only way she can do that is by catching them and allowing her body to fight off the infection. Every time she does this, her immune system becomes that little bit stronger. I'm not suggesting you take her to crowded places and purposefully infect her, but equally don't coop her up at home. Just be sensible and live a normal life.

Croup

This is another common virus that usually affects babies and children from six months to three years. The virus causes the voice box (larynx) and airways to the lungs (trachea) to swell, making it difficult to breathe. In adults the same illness is called laryngitis.

Croup causes a very distinctive barking cough. It mainly affects children in the middle of the night.

Other symptoms include:

- Sore throat
- Runny nose
- Fever – 38°C (100.4°F) or higher
- Loud, high-pitched rasping sound when breathing

It generally lasts for a maximum of four to six days.

Treatment

Take your baby to the doctor for a diagnosis, but treatment at home until symptoms pass is usually the best option unless the croup develops and your baby seems to have trouble breathing.

- Infant paracetamol/ibuprofen
- Lots of TLC
- Extra fluids as the bark-like cough is likely to make her thirsty

Thrush in babies

Symptoms in babies can include one or more white spot or particles in and around the baby's mouth. These may look yellow or cream coloured, like curd or cottage cheese. They can also join together to make larger plagues. You may see patches on:

- Her gums
- The roof of her mouth
- Inside her cheeks

You will find that you can easily rub the patches off but the tissue underneath will be red and raw and may also bleed a little. The patches may not seem to bother her but if they are sore she may be reluctant to feed.

Other signs and symptoms are:

- A whitish sheen to the saliva
- Fussiness at the breast – keeps detaching
- Refusing the breast
- Clicking sounds during feeding
- Poor weight gain
- Nappy rash
- Some babies may dribble more saliva than normal

Oral thrush affects about 1 in 20 babies and is most common in babies around four weeks, although older babies can get it too.

Treatment
Many cases of oral thrush clear up in a few days without treatment, but it is wise to see your GP if you suspect that your baby does have thrush to be advised on treatment depending on the severity of it.

Thrush in mothers
If you are breastfeeding it is possible that your baby will pass the infection on to you, which will affect your nipples or breasts; this is known as nipple thrush.

Symptoms include:

- Pain while feeding which may continue after the feed has finished
- Cracked, flaky or sensitive nipples or areolas (dark skin around the nipple)

Treatment
Again, see your GP if you think that you may have nipple thrush.

Sickness and diarrhoea

Diarrhoea, again, is caused by a virus and spreads like wildfire through households once one family member catches it. This is the one bug I always try to avoid at all costs. I'm usually pretty relaxed about meeting up with friends if they or their children have coughs or colds, but if I know someone in their house has recently had diarrhoea and vomiting then I will avoid them for a few days to try to reduce the risk of the bug entering our house!

It will be pretty obvious if your baby has caught a diarrhoea and sickness bug. Even if she is usually a sicky baby, the vomit produced when they have a bug is usually in vast quantities. She may have diarrhoea with the vomiting or she may only have one or the other. Other symptoms to indicate she has this type of bug are:

- Refusal to feed, and the milk or solids that she does take come straight back out again in the form of vomit or loose nappies
- Not being interested in feeding again despite having an empty tummy
- Possible temperature – over 38°C (10.4°F)
- Being clingy, lethargic and just wanting cuddles

Treatment
Generally diarrhoea and vomiting clears up on its own without treatment from a doctor within 24–48 hours. Hygiene is of the utmost importance while anyone in the house has diarrhoea and

vomiting to prevent the risk of it spreading. Hand washing should be done with anti-bacterial soap, and lots of bleach products should be used in toilets and sinks which come into contact with the liquid produced from both ends! You also need to wash all clothing and bedding that is soiled on a 60°C wash to kill germs.

The treatment for diarrhoea and vomiting in older children and adults is to not eat anything at all, in order to give the body time to fight off the bug without 'feeding' it. Specifically, it is a good idea to avoid dairy and milk products during the illness and for a couple of days afterwards, as these are thought to make the bug worse. Obviously, in small babies avoiding milk is virtually impossible – particularly if they haven't ever been introduced to solids yet.

Breast or formula milk is their food as well as hydration, so you cannot stop feeding them completely. However, you will likely find that your baby will want to feed less anyway, because she is feeling unwell. If breastfeeding, just feed her little and often to keep her hydrated. Giving her big feeds every few hours is more likely to make her sick as it will be too much for her tummy to cope with. Go with the flow in terms of feeding and sleep while she is ill, and once better you can aim to get her back into her normal routine again.

If she is formula fed and doesn't seem to be tolerating her feeds, then you can try offering her half-strength feeds to see if she manages to keep those down instead. A half-strength feed won't be as rich for her tummy while she has a bug, and the extra water the feed contains means you will be giving her added hydration too when she needs it most. As she begins to improve you can put her feeds back to normal again. It is advisable if you have been half strengthening all of her feeds, to do this gradually, so begin by moving every other feed up to full strength. If she tolerates these without being sick, then you can make the remaining feeds back up to full strength as normal.

It is very normal for the diarrhoea to linger for a few days or even a week or two, even after the sickness has cleared up. This is because the bug is not able to be 'starved out of their system' in a baby like it is with an older child or adult, because she will still continue at least some of her milk feeds while she has the bug.

Although this bug usually clears up on its own, if you are at all worried about your baby, then take her to see your GP. Symptoms to watch out for that need a doctor's attention are:

- Sunken fontanelle and eyes – a sign of dehydration
- Loose, pale or mottled skin
- Hardly passing any urine
- Cold hands and feet

Cradle cap

This is the name given to the yellowish, greasy scaly patches that appear on the scalp of babies. It usually develops at some point within the first two months of your baby being born. It is not contagious and is not due to poor health or hygiene. Exactly what causes it is not clear, but it may be linked to the sebaceous glands, which are glands in the skin that produce an oily substance called sebum. In some very lucky babies it will only last a few weeks or months, but for most it can linger around for up to one to two years.

Treatment

There is no specific treatment advisable by a doctor for cradle cap. Gently washing your baby's hair and scalp may prevent a build up of scales – there are shampoos available for this purpose that can be bought at the supermarket – however they don't make your baby's head smell too sweet! Gently massaging olive oil into the scalp at night after a bath can also help to loosen the crust. This will then become flaky and then fall out, although sometimes the hair can come away with the flakes. It is important not to pick at the scales as this can cause infection.

Blocked milk ducts

This is very common, particularly in the first few days of engorgement when your breast milk comes in just after your baby is born. You may feel various lumps in one or both breasts and also sometimes in your armpit.

Your breasts go into overdrive in the first few days and try to produce as much milk as possible. This is sometimes too much for the milk ducts to cope with and they become blocked. This is extremely painful. To relieve symptoms it is important that your baby is encouraged to empty the breast regularly. If your baby doesn't take a big feed and your breasts still feel very full, lumpy and engorged then you can use a breast pump to express any excess milk off to give you some relief. This can be stored in the fridge or freezer and used at a later date.

Treatment

Massaging where the lump is will also help massively. Massage the lump in a stroking motion towards the nipple. This will help to unblock the duct and encourage a better flow. You can do this while feeding and in between feeds too. Engorgement and blocked ducts are more common in the first couple of weeks when your milk supply is much higher, but can happen at any time. If you also feel ill with the painful breasts or are suffering from other symptoms then you may have mastitis (see opposite).

Both blocked milk ducts and mastitis can also affect mothers who don't breastfeed and whose babies have had formula from birth. In this instance I would advise against expressing the milk off because that will just encourage your breasts to keep producing milk that you don't want to use. Massage your breasts as directed above or take a hot bath or shower with flannels on your breasts to relieve symptoms. See your doctor if you think you may have mastitis.

Mastitis

Mastitis is caused by milk stasis and happens when milk builds up in your breasts because it is being made faster than it is being removed. Milk stasis can happen when your baby isn't emptying your breasts well when she feeds – this can be because she isn't latched on properly.

Mastitis usually only affects one breast and symptoms can develop quickly. These include:

- A red swollen area on your breast that may feel hot and painful to touch
- An area of hardness on your breast
- A burning pain in your breast that may be continuous or may only occur when you are breastfeeding
- Nipple discharge – which may be white or may contain streaks of blood

Over half of women with mastitis may also experience flu-like symptoms such as:

- Aches
- High temperature of 38°C (100.4°F) or above
- Shivering and chills
- Tiredness
- Feeling generally unwell

Visit your GP immediately if you experience these symptoms and you also have a red tender area on your breast.

Treatment

Mastitis is not usually serious but advice and prompt treatment may be needed to stop it getting worse. Your doctor may prescribe antibiotics.

Some self-help treatments to help relieve symptoms are:

- Express off any excess milk your baby doesn't take at a feed to stop your breasts being so full and engorged and therefore painful.
- Check your baby is latched on correctly. Try different feeding positions if you are not sure.
- Try warm flannels or a warm bath or shower to help relieve the pain, although some mothers prefer cold flannels.
- Gently massage your breasts to help the milk flow better as your baby feeds.
- Painkillers can be taken at your doctor's advice

Post-natal depression (PND)

There are many feelings, both good and bad, that come with the birth of your baby. The baby blues all mothers tend to experience within the first two weeks after giving birth are very normal and connected with your hormones rather than anything else.

Many new mothers feel overwhelmed, stressed and in need of a break at some point when their baby is small. Recognising when this feeling, as well as others, has developed into something more is difficult. Below is a list of the differences between feelings felt by every new mum that are normal and feelings or symptoms that are likely to be signs that you are suffering from post-natal depression and need to see and speak to your health visitor or doctor.

The information below is taken from an article written by Kate Kripke of The Postpartum Wellness Center of Boulder. She is a licensed clinical social worker and runs a clinic specialising in the prevention and treatment of perinatal mood disorders, including PND and anxiety. In my opinion the details below give a clear indication to mothers about what are normal feelings and what feelings are related to PND.

Healthy and normal

- *Some feelings of overwhelm and anxiety that decrease with reassurance.*
- *Some 'escapist fantasies' (a desire to run away) that occur when the logistics of motherhood are challenging but go away when your baby is soothed, when you are rested and when you are validated.*
- *Fears about harm coming to your baby that come and go, that you know are not realistic, but that decrease as your experience and comfort with motherhood grows.*
- *Sleeplessness that occurs from caring for your baby at night, while still having the ability to sleep when your baby is sleeping, or when given the option to rest.*
- *Fatigue that comes from late night feedings and interrupted sleep.*
- *Some feelings of frustration towards your partner regarding differences in parenting choices or differing roles.*
- *Moments of sadness, disappointment or anger towards your parents when reminded of the ways that you were parented, but the ability to hold insight and perspective regarding your own relationship with your baby.*
- *Feelings of isolation that are caused by the increased time spent with your baby, especially when newborn, but also a desire and motivation to connect with others.*
- *Uncertainty that comes with this new job and building confidence that comes with time.*
- *A hesitancy and worry that comes with allowing others to care for your baby, but a willingness to do this when you are in need of a break.*
- *A decrease in eating that is caused by the busyness of being a new mum.*
- *Temporary body aches and pains that are a result of childbirth and/or feeding.*

- Acknowledgement of the challenge that comes with new mother-hood, but also the ability to look forward to things getting easier.
- Increases in energy that comes with increases in sleep.
- Feelings of worry about your baby's ability to latch or feed as you hoped that decreases with feeding improvement, or that shift when a new feeding option is chosen.
- Vulnerable feelings that come and go but that do not alter the way that you think about yourself.

PND that requires support

- Feeling anxious and overwhelmed most of the time – an anxiety that doesn't go away with reassurance.
- Feelings of regret over becoming a mum that do not seem to go away.
- Repetitive and intrusive thoughts of harm coming to your baby that cause great distress, and that impact on your ability to care for your baby.
- Sleeplessness that occurs due to 'monkey brain' – anxious thoughts that will not go away.
- A deep fatigue that is not alleviated with rest and/or a desire to remain in bed all day.
- Relentless feelings of anger and rage towards your partner and/or others.
- Resurfacing memories about your own early childhood that cause great distress, anxiety or sadness.
- Loneliness and isolation that occur while also pulling away from those who care about you; a lack of desire or motivation to connect with others.
- Persistent feelings that you are not a good mum or you are not good at doing motherly things, even despite validation or reassurance from others.

- *Feelings that your baby does not 'like you' because she cries or is not feeding well*
- *Unrelenting anxiety about having others help care for your baby, and a deep fear and inability to let go of some of this control.*
- *Thoughts of hurting yourself.*
- *Lacking appetite or a need to keep eating despite being full.*
- *Body aches and pains with no apparent cause.*
- *Never-ending feelings that you will never feel better.*
- *Sudden increase in energy that occurs despite a decrease in sleep; this may or may not include seeing or hearing things that aren't really there.*
- *A general feeling of 'not feeling like yourself.'*

Post-natal depression is just one of the many postpartum mood disorders. Other categories include: postpartum anxiety, postpartum panic disorder, postpartum OCD, postpartum PTSD, and postpartum psychosis (affecting 0.1–0.2 per cent of new mums, many of whom have a prior history of bipolar disorder). They can develop anytime within the first 12 months after your baby's birth.

Every single postpartum mood disorder, including postpartum psychosis, is treatable, and women who seek help and follow treatment recommendations do get better.

For more information visit www.postpartumprogress.com.

Treatment

You should seek treatment if any uncomfortable or vulnerable feelings persist for longer than two to three weeks, especially when they interfere with your ability to meet your basic needs and/or live your life as you would like to.

Motherhood is challenging for all of us, but it should not be consistently distressing or miserable. If you are finding yourself wondering if what you are struggling with is 'normal', a good question to ask yourself is 'Is this normal for me when I am well?' If it is not, then there is help waiting – you do not need to suffer through the symptoms of PND. Help is available and it is important that you ask for it if you are feeling overwhelmed, as, even though you may not feel like things will ever improve, they most definitely will if you seek help.

Turned-in foot (pigeon-toed)

If your baby was born with one or both feet turned inwards, it is likely your paediatrician will have noticed it before you left the hospital. If they didn't then it is a good idea to mention it to your midwife, health visitor or doctor. While sometimes it can be genetic, it is very common for it to develop because of the cramped position your baby was in during her time in the womb.

Treatment

The usual advice is to gently massage her foot back the correct way on a daily basis. If breastfeeding, this can be a great time to do it if you have a spare hand. Your doctor/midwife will show you how to do this correctly. Most cases usually resolve themselves by the time a baby is six months old.

If it doesn't begin to improve or you think it is getting worse, then go back to your doctor and ask to be referred to a specialist. Severe pigeon-toeing can resemble club foot or accompany other foot problems that need to be addressed.

My third child had her left foot turned in when she was born, due to her cramped position in the womb. She was my only baby that this happened to, and my previous two babies had been fine. We were shown how to massage and manipulate her foot each day to encourage it to straighten out, and by the time she was three months old her foot was fine and looked normal again.

Cleft Palate

A cleft lip and palate is the most common facial birth defect in the UK. One in every 700 babies is born with a cleft. The type of cleft and how severe it is can vary widely between children. Approximately half of all affected babies are born with a cleft lip and palate, a third with a cleft only and 1 in 10 has a cleft lip only or a sub-mucous cleft (see below). A cleft is a gap or split in either the upper lip or the roof of the mouth (palate) or sometimes both. It occurs when separate areas of the face do not join together properly when a baby is developing during pregnancy. The face and upper lip develop during the fifth to ninth week of pregnancy. Most cleft problems can either be picked up at the routine 20-week scan or soon after birth. However a sub-mucous cleft, where the cleft is hidden in the lining of the roof of the mouth, may not be detected for months or even years.

The exact cause of clefts is not known, although evidence suggests they are caused by a combination of genetics and environmental factors. Cleft lips can occur on their own or are sometimes part of a wider series of birth defects. A cleft can lead to feeding, speech, hearing problems, ear infections, dental decay, jaw development problems and psychosocial issues if not treated.

Treatment

Surgery is the usual treatment for cleft lip and palate, with good results. After treatment most children have a normal appearance with minimal scarring and normal speech. All types of treatment for cleft lip and palate are available on the NHS. A long-term structural care plan from a team of cleft specialists is usually needed to help children born with clefts.

Cranial osteopathy to treat babies after traumatic labours

This is a gentle and safe treatment where very specific light pressure is applied to the skull where necessary, to assist and encourage your baby's body to naturally release stress and tension. Being born can be a very traumatic experience for some babies, particularly if you have had an assisted delivery where ventouse or forceps have been used.

With some babies, parents have been recommended to try cranial osteopathy. Reactions to treatments are variable – often the baby is very relaxed afterwards and sleeps well. Others have a burst of energy after treatment, usually followed by a good night's sleep. Many parents agree that this treatment can be helpful, but few would say it is a miracle cure.

You can search for details of your local osteopath by visiting www.osteopathy.org.uk

Tongue tie

Tongue tie is a birth defect that affects 3–10 per cent of newborn babies. It is more common in boys than girls and appears to be genetically passed down. Normally the tongue is loosely attached to the base of the mouth with a piece of skin called the frenulum. In babies with tongue tie this piece of skin is much shorter and holds the tongue down, restricting the movement. It doesn't always cause problems and sometimes the skin anchoring the tongue may be so thin that it soon breaks, solving the problem. However in some cases it can be more severe and require treatment.

Tongue tie can be hard to diagnose in newborns. It is important to contact your doctor if you are worried that your baby may be affected.

Signs of tongue tie in a breastfed baby are:

- The baby has difficulty latching on to the nipple
- She often loses suction while feeding and sucks in air
- She makes a clicking sound while feeding
- The mother has sore nipples during and after feeding
- The mother has squashed nipples after breastfeeding
- The mother has white compression marks on the nipple after breastfeeding
- The baby fails to gain weight

A tongue-tied baby may also find bottle-feeding hard. They cannot form a seal around the teat of the bottle, so milk leaks out as they suck. Air can sometimes get in and is swallowed, causing the baby to become windy and irritable. A bottle-fed baby is also likely to make the clicking sound when feeding too.

Treatment

Snipping the skin to free the tongue is known as tongue-tie division or frenuloplasty. It is a simple and painless procedure that usually resolves the feeding problems mentioned above straight away. In babies younger than eight months, division of tongue tie is usually performed without any anaesthetic or with just a local anaesthetic that numbs the skin. A general anaesthetic is usually needed for older babies, which means they will be put to sleep before the procedure. The baby's head is held securely and sharp scissors are used to snip the piece of skin. This only takes a few seconds and the baby won't feel much pain. Some babies sleep through it while others just cry for a few seconds. There should be little or no blood loss and you can start feeding your baby immediately. A white patch may form under the tongue, which takes 24–48 hours to heal but does not bother the baby.

Red/sore bottom

This is a very common occurrence for all babies and some will seem to suffer from it more regularly than others. Teething, fragranced or perfumed wet wipes or having a soiled nappy on for too long can all cause your baby to get a red or sore bottom.

Treatment

'Air time' is the best form of treatment, which involves allowing your baby to have her nappy off for regular periods during the day. This will improve the rash or redness in the fastest time. You can lay her on a towel to catch any 'accidents' she has while not wearing her nappy. When it is time to put it back on again, then apply a nappy-rash cream. In my experience Sudocrem or Metanium seem to be the most effective. Less is more – do not be tempted to apply lashings of cream. This will possibly make her bottom even more sore, as the excess cream that doesn't sink into the skin will sit on the surface of her nappy and act as a barrier, preventing it from absorbing the urine that your baby does. This urine will then sit on her skin and makes her even sorer.

See your GP if you have tried all of the above and it doesn't seem to be improving, as your baby may have thrush that needs treating with a different cream from your doctor.

Conjunctivitis

Conjunctivitis is redness and inflammation of the thin layer of tissue that covers the front of the eye (conjunctiva) and is very common. Other symptoms include itchiness and watering of the eyes and sometimes a sticky coating on the eyelashes. It can affect one or both eyes. The most obvious symptom is having green 'goo' in the corners of the eye. If both eyes are affected, then use a separate piece of cotton wool and water to wipe it away. Always wipe from the inside to the outside of the eye. If it comes back fairly quickly then it's likely your baby has infected conjunctivitis that requires antibiotic treatment.

Treatment

In many cases conjunctivitis doesn't require treatment in older children and adults, as symptoms usually clear up within a couple of weeks. However, if you think your baby or child has infected conjunctivitis then see your GP straight away for treatment. It is very contagious, so hand-washing after touching your baby's eyes and using separate towels from the infected people, will prevent the risk of it spreading to other members of the family.

Hernia

There are two types of hernia that can occur in babies: an umbilical hernia and an inguinal hernia.

Umbilical hernia

An umbilical hernia appears as a lump near the navel (belly button) that may get bigger when your baby laughs, cries, coughs or goes to the toilet. It may also shrink when she is relaxed or lying down.

During pregnancy the umbilical cord passes through an opening in the baby's abdominal wall. This opening should close before birth, but in some cases the muscles do not seal completely. This leaves a weak spot in the surrounding muscle wall (abdominal wall). An umbilical hernia can develop when fatty tissue or a part of the bowel pokes through into an area near the navel.

Umbilical hernias are very common and affect 10 per cent of infants and young children. They are particularly common in babies born prematurely. An umbilical hernia is not painful, and in 85 per cent of cases the umbilical hernia goes back in and the muscles release before your child's first birthday.

Treatment

If the umbilical hernia is large or has not disappeared by the time a child reaches four years old, an umbilical repair is an option. Your doctor will advise you to wait until this age before considering operating though, as it is not an essential procedure unless there are other complications.

An umbilical repair is a routine and simple procedure to push the bulge back in place and strengthen the abdominal wall. A general anaesthetic will be used on your child and the operation should only last around 30 minutes. The weak spot is usually closed with stitches and after the operation the bulge will disappear and the belly button should look normal.

Inguinal hernia

An inguinal hernia is where a small hole has developed in the muscle of a baby's groin. Some of the intestine then pokes out through this hole. The intestine in the hernia usually moves in and out of the hernia quite easily. Sometimes the intestine may get stuck in the hernia leading to blockage of, and possibly damage to the intestine or to the blood vessels to the testicle. If this happens then emergency surgery is needed as the intestine or testicle can be damaged. Doctors usually plan to fix the hernia before this happens though. Inguinal (groin) hernias are quite common and happen in around one in six premature baby boys. These hernias usually require an operation before they reach an emergency state.

Treatment

Under anaesthetic, a cut will be made in the baby's groin. The hole in the muscle will be repaired with stitches and the skin closed with stitches under the surface. A small dressing may be applied, and local anaesthetic will also be used to numb the skin so as to reduce any pain the baby may be in after surgery. Infant paracetamol can be given for pain relief as directed by your doctor.

Birthmarks

This is a coloured mark that develops on or just under the skin before or soon after birth, and affects one in three babies. Some fade with time, others become more prominent and obvious and permanent unless removed. Most are harmless and require no treatment. Most common are the little pink and red marks that people refer to as 'stork marks'. These marks appear V-shaped on the forehead and upper eyelids, and will gradually fade, although it can sometimes take a few months. Marks on the nape of the neck can last much longer but are usually covered by hair anyway. Strawberry marks are quite common too. They're dark red and slightly raised and sometimes appear a few days after birth and gradually get bigger. They may take a while to go away, and can grow quite big before they do, but most begin to reduce in size and then eventually disappear.

Immunisations

Having your baby vaccinated against certain illnesses and diseases is a personal choice that each parent is entitled to make based on any research they decide to do. Below is a checklist of the vaccines that are routinely offered to everyone in the UK for free on the NHS and at the age at which they should ideally be given. Each vaccination is given as a single injection into the muscle of the thigh or upper arm.

Immunisations available on the NHS

Two months (eight weeks). *Two separate needles are given.*

1: *5-in-1 Dtap/IPV/Hib*
   This single jab contains vaccines to protect against five separate diseases: diphtheria, tetanus, pertussis (whooping cough), polio and haemophilus influenza type B (Hib – a bacterial infection that can cause severe pneumonia or meningitis in young children).

2: *Pneumococcal infection*

Three months *(12 weeks, or four weeks after the first vaccination). Two separate needles are given.*

1: *5-in-1 second dose (details as above)*

2: *Meningitis C*

Four months *(16 weeks, or four weeks after the second vaccination). Three separate needles are given.*

1: *5-in-1 third dose (details as above)*

2: *Pneumococcal infection second dose*

3: *Meningitis C second dose*

12–13 months. *Three needles are given.*

1: *Hib/meningitis C booster given as a single jab containing meningitis C third dose and Hib fourth dose*

2: *MMR (measles, mumps and rubella) given as a single jab*

3: *Pneumococcal infection third dose*

Three years + four months, or soon after. *Two needles are given.*
1: *MMR second dose*
2: *4-in-1 pre-school booster (Dtap/IPV) given as a single jab containing vaccines against diphtheria, tetanus, pertussis and polio*

12–13 years *(girls only)*
HPV vaccine, which protects against cervical cancer, given as three jabs within six months

13–18 years
3-in-1 teenage booster given as a single jab which contains vaccines against diphtheria, tetanus and polio

Whooping cough is now being offered as a vaccine to expectant mothers. As there has been a rise in whooping cough cases in babies too young to have started their routine vaccination, immunising the expectant mother is one way to prevent babies catching it once they're born.

Until 2005 the BCG injection (TB) was given to school children when they were 15 years old, but this has been stopped because so many areas in the UK now have such low TB rates. Instead, the health authorities are targeting high-rate areas, where they are vaccinating babies. So if your baby is offered a BCG jab it is probably because you live in an area where the TB rate is high, often an inner-city area.

Babies will also be offered the BCG jab if their parents or grandparents have lived in an area with a high TB rate such as South Asia and some parts of Africa. If you think that there is a chance that your baby may be at risk then speak to your health visitor about having your baby vaccinated. However, unless there is someone living in your household who has TB, your baby is almost certainly safe because this disease is very difficult to catch.

8

Developmental stages from birth to 24 months

Babies vary greatly in the ages that they do various physical things like rolling, crawling, walking and even cutting teeth. To a certain extent you as a parent have to trust your instincts as to whether they seem to be developing normally or not. People will tell you not to compare your baby to friends' babies, but it is only natural to do this, particularly if the babies are of similar ages. However, it's good to try to realise that babies don't all develop in the same way. Some babies skip the rolling stage completely. Some never crawl and go straight on to the walking stage. Every baby has their own personality and will develop at their own rate. As long as you, or your doctor or health visitor, have not noticed any physical abnormalities that may hinder her development, then just be patient and she will reach her milestones at her own speed.

Even siblings will do things at completely different ages. My own three children were all very different. My firstborn crawled at nine months, walked at 11 months and we could hold a two-way conversation with him speaking clearly by 18 months. My second son didn't crawl until he was 11 and a half months, didn't walk until he was almost 17 months and barely said a word (although understood what was said to him) until he was over two years old. My third child was different again – she crawled at 11 months, walked at 15 months and was saying lots of simple words and stringing a few two-word blocks together by 17 months.

Below I have compiled a month-by-month guide on what your baby may be capable of, which is taken from the www.babycentre. co.uk. Underneath I have suggested what you can do to encourage further development to the next stage, and the types of toys she may be interested in. The charts are purely a guide and even if your child isn't doing certain things at a certain age then you probably have nothing to worry about and she will soon catch up or be excelling and concentrating on other areas. A baby who is slower to move physically may be babbling, understanding and learning new words faster than another baby who can crawl across a room in seconds! They are all different and generally at the same level by the time they begin school.

Newborn to one month

- Will display the newborn reflexes, as described in Chapter 3
- Turns towards bright lights
- Can focus clearly up to 20–25cm (8–10in) away (breast to face distance)
- Can see simple, high-contrast patterns that are further away
- Is startled by loud noises
- Can lift her head briefly while on her tummy
- Has equal movements of arms and legs on both sides of her body. For example, she shouldn't move one arm or leg much more than the other – if she can, this could be a sign of weakness or injury
- Will spontaneously smile at random times, even while asleep. This smile is present from birth and different to the 'social smile' that happens in response to being talked or sung to later on

What you can do

- Talk to your baby all the time about anything and everything, even if you are not holding her, and encourage your partner to do the same. She will be reassured and soothed by the comfort of hearing your voice that she has become so used to while inside you, particularly when she is upset.

- Encourage a brief tummy time each day – if you start this from newborn your baby is more likely to enjoy it. Tummy time helps to strengthen the baby's neck, back and trunk muscles. Babies need strong muscle groups in order to sit, crawl and walk. It can also help avoid flat head syndrome, as babies who spend too much time on their backs or in baby recliners can develop flat spots on their heads (see page 189). Visual development will also be aided as your baby learns to track movement and focus on objects.

Toys
- At this stage your baby will be unable to hold any toys to do anything with. She will grasp anything you place in her hand but won't connect her hand and mouth together to be able to see what she is holding.
- She will enjoy looking at bold black and white pictures or objects, and you may find her staring at high-contrast pictures you have on the walls or even your ceiling beams if you live in an old house.
- She will enjoy hearing music, and toys that light up may catch her attention too for a short time.

At one month
Mastered skills (that most babies can do)
- Responds to sound
- Stares at faces
- Lifts head

Emerging skills (that half of children can do)
- Follows objects
- Makes 'ooh' and 'ahhh' sounds
- Can see black and white patterns

Advanced skills (that a few babies will be able to do)
- Smiles socially in response to being talked to or sung to
- Laughs
- Can hold head at 45° angle

Toys and parental encouragement
To continue everything suggested above for a newborn. Talk, sing and engage with your baby as much as possible. She will learn to smile in response to copying you. Silly voices and over-the-top, big cheesy smiles will encourage her to mimic what you are doing.

At two months
Mastered skills
- Vocalises, gurgles and coos
- Follows objects
- Holds head up for short periods

Emerging skills
- Smiles in response to another person. Laughs
- Holds head at 45° angle
- Movements become smoother

Advanced skills
- Holds head steady
- Bears weight on legs
- May lift head and shoulder – mini push up

Toys and parental encouragement
Continue talking and singing to your baby. Coo and gurgle, making the same noises she does as she begins to vocalise – this will encourage her to do it even more, as she will love to engage with you.

Encourage daily tummy time.

She may now begin to also enjoy lying under a baby gym for short periods of time and looking up at the toys, or lights and sounds if you have a musical one.

At three months
Mastered skills
- Laughs
- Holds head steady
- Recognises your face and smell and is comforted by it when upset

Emerging skills
- Squeals, gurgles and coos
- Recognises your voice
- Does mini push ups (lifts head and shoulders)

Advanced skills
- Turns towards loud sounds
- Can bring hands together and may bat at toys
- Can roll over

Toys and parental encouragement
She will really begin to enjoy holding toys now, and gradually get the idea of moving her hand to her mouth to chew on the toy as her hand–eye coordination improves on a daily basis. Try to pick lighter rattles at this stage, as she will end up hitting herself with the rattle fairly frequently to begin with, as she is learning how to control her movements and is less likely to hurt herself with a smaller rattle. It will also be easier for her to grasp.

She will also enjoy lying under her baby gym and rolling from side to side and waving her arms and legs around – even if she can't actually roll over properly yet.

Continue to encourage daily tummy time.

At four months
Mastered skills
- Holds head up steadily
- Can bear weight on legs
- Coos when you talk to her, as if talking back

Emerging skills
- Can grasp a toy
- Reaches out for objects
- Can roll over

Advanced skills
- Imitates speech sounds: baba, dada
- May cut first tooth

Toys and parental encouragement
She will be very interested in everything around her now. She will be aware of different environments and enjoy even changing from one room to another if she is beginning to get bored at 'playing' in one particular place. She will enjoy a variety of toys too and be developing good hand–eye coordination to be able to move objects to her mouth to chew. You may want to try a mother-and-baby group at this stage if you haven't already, as it is something that will benefit both of you.

At five months
Mastered skills
- Can distinguish between bold colours
- Can roll over
- Amuses herself by playing with hands and feet

Emerging skills
- Turns towards new sounds
- Recognises own name
- May be ready for solids

Advanced skills
- May sit momentarily without support
- Mouths objects
- Stranger anxiety may now begin

Toys and parental encouragement
She may enjoy blow-up support rings now to encourage her ability to learn to sit up. A Bumbo seat is also another good item that will help strengthen her back muscles and encourage her to sit unaided eventually. (Both of these should only be used on flat surfaces.) She will begin to enjoy musical toys more, especially ones that make noises when she does certain things. While at home, make sure you go off and do things around the house as she plays safely somewhere on her mat. This will prevent her becoming anxious about you leaving the room as she gets older, as she will have learnt from a young age that you always return. Check on her every five minutes, though, to make sure all is well, and make a point of chatting to her each time you do, so that she is reassured she is not alone.

At six months
Mastered skills
- Turns towards sounds and voices
- Imitates sounds – blows bubbles or raspberries
- Rolls in both directions

Emerging skills
- Sits without support
- Reaches for objects and mouths them
- Is ready for solids

Advanced skills
- May lunge forward or start crawling
- May jabber or combine syllables
- May drag objects towards herself

Toys and parental encouragement

At this stage your baby may enjoy a door bouncer or something like an activity centre, where she is able to bear her weight and jump up and down. You should also still be encouraging and teaching her how to learn to sit up unaided by sitting her up with support. As she gets increasingly better at this, you can just put a variety of cushions and pillows all around her to break her fall if she does decide to topple over. Even when babies seem to have 'cracked' learning to sit up unaided, they still tend to topple over every now and again, so it is safer to have the pillow ready to catch them! Don't worry if she isn't rolling – many babies do not roll until much later or even at all. None of my babies rolled until they were closer to eight months!

At seven months
Mastered skills
- Sits without support
- Reaches for things with a sweeping motion
- Imitates speech sounds (babbles)

Emerging skills
- Combines syllables into word-like sounds
- Begins to crawl or lunges forward

Advanced skills
- Stands while holding on to something
- Waves goodbye
- Bangs objects together

Toys and parental encouragement

Sing songs and repeat things like showing her how to wave bye-bye and clapping her hands. The more you do this and repeat, the quicker she will learn to pick the action up and do it herself.

Put objects slightly further away from her if you notice she is trying to reach out for things. This will make her more determined and motivated to move to get them.

Read first-word books together and repeat things, like animal names in particular with the sounds they make, over and over. Use very simple terms like:

Sheep – baa. What does the sheep say?... Baa.

Cow – moo. What does the cow say?... Moo

If you repeat things like this on a daily basis your baby will learn very quickly. All three of my children could make between five and ten animal noises when prompted by the age of ten months.

At eight months
Mastered skills
- Says 'Dada' and 'Mama' to both parents – isn't specific
- Begins to crawl
- Passes objects from hand to hand

Emerging skills
- Stands while holding on to something
- Crawls well
- Points at objects

Advanced skills
- Pulls self to standing position and 'cruises' around the furniture while holding on
- Picks things up with pincer grasp (thumb and finger)
- Indicates wants with gestures

Toys and parental encouragement
Continue everything as suggested in the seven-month age group. If she is already showing signs of standing and wanting to walk then a baby walker is another option she may enjoy to get herself around the house. If she's already crawling or moving around by other means – rolling or bottom shuffling – she will have her own means of moving and won't like the restriction of a baby walker that she sits inside; she will prefer a free-standing one that you

can help her to push along. The wooden ones or the tripod-type plastic ones are the sturdiest.

Smaller finger foods to encourage development of her pincer grasp will help her physical development too.

At nine months
Mastered skills
- Combines syllables into word-like sounds
- Stands while holding on to something

Emerging skills
- Uses pincer grasp to pick up objects
- Cruises around the furniture
- Bangs objects together

Advanced skills
- Plays pat-a-cake (can clap hands when prompted)
- Says 'Dada' and 'Mama' to the right person

Toys and parental encouragement
Continue everything you are doing. Read together, sing to her and use actions with the songs to teach her new things. She may enjoy stacking objects or bricks at this stage and also banging the bricks together or any other two objects she picks up at the same time. Separation anxiety can begin anytime from now, so if she isn't used to a variety of environments while with you, she will begin to get more anxious from this point onwards in new situations. If you are considering a childminder or nursery as a form of childcare when returning to work, it is better to start it now before her anxiety gets to the point where she will be upset at being left. She is then more likely to adapt and settle into the new arrangement very quickly and easily.

At 10 months
Mastered skills
- Waves bye-bye
- Picks things up with pincer grasp
- Crawls well
- Cruises around the furniture

Emerging skills
- Says 'Dada' and 'Mama' to the right person
- Responds to her name and understands the word 'no'
- Indicates wants with gestures

Advanced skills
- Drinks from a cup
- Stands alone for a couple of seconds
- Puts objects into a container

Toys and parental encouragement
Continue the use of baby walkers to encourage independent walking as she gains confidence. She will also enjoy holding on to your fingers and walking round the house like this. As her stability improves you will be able to reduce to just holding one of her hands with yours and then eventually letting go for short periods of time. If she is still yet to crawl, then putting her in the required starting position and encouraging her to move by putting objects slightly out of reach will motivate her to move.

At 11 months
Mastered skills
- Says 'Dada' and 'Mama' to the right person
- Plays 'pat-a-cake'
- Stands alone

Emerging skills
- Imitates others' activities
- Puts objects into a container
- Understands simple instructions ('Go and get your cup', 'Put that in the bin', etc.)

Advanced skills
- Drinks from a cup
- Says one other word beside 'Mama' and 'Dada'
- Stoops to bending down from a standing position

Toys and parental encouragement
Continue activities discussed at 10 months. Encourage her understanding by giving her simple instructions to follow: 'Go and get your ball', 'Put this in the bin', etc. on a daily basis. She will enjoy having a saucepan or bowl to play with and putting things in it and then taking them all out again repeatedly. Showing her what to do will encourage her to mimic and copy your actions.

At 12 months
Mastered skills
- Imitates others' activities
- Jabbers word-like sounds
- Indicates wants with gestures

Emerging skills
- Says one other word beside 'Mama' and 'Dada'
- Takes a few steps
- Understands and responds to simple instructions

Advanced skills
- Scribbles with a crayon
- Walks well
- Says two other words beside 'Mama' and 'Dada'

Toys and parental encouragement
Continue to encourage development of her physical and verbal skills by giving her opportunities to practise walking and vocalising on a daily basis. The more you chat to her, the more she will learn. She will enjoy copying things you are doing – if you are cooking then give her a saucepan and a spoon to mix. She may also enjoy loading and unloading the washing machine, and various other household chores, which you can chat to her about as you are doing them, giving her instructions which she will quickly learn as you do.

At 13 months
Mastered skills
- Uses two words skilfully (e.g., hello and bye-bye)
- Bends over and picks up objects
- Stands alone

Emerging skills
- Enjoys gazing at her reflection
- Drinks from a cup
- Plays peek-a-boo

Advanced skills
- Combines words and gestures to make needs known
- Tries to lift heavy things
- Rolls a ball back and forth

Toys and parental encouragement
Continue as above for 12-month age group, giving her opportunities to improve skills.

At 14 months
Mastered skills
- Finger feeds

- Empties containers of contents
- Imitates others

Emerging skills
- Toddles well
- Imitates games
- Points to a body part when asked

Advanced skills
- Uses spoon or fork
- Matches lids with appropriate containers, e.g., pots and pans
- Pushes and pulls toys while walking

Toys and parental encouragement
She will enjoy simple games where she can copy something you are doing. She will also like putting items in containers so that she can do her favourite part of emptying them all out again! This is a good stage to encourage her to tidy away her toys once she finishes with them, as she will be so eager to do it. If taught to tidy away from a young age you stand more chance of her continuing this good habit as she gets older.

At 15 months
Mastered skills
- Plays with a ball
- Vocab has increased up to five words
- Can walk backwards

Emerging skills
- Can draw a line
- Runs well
- Adopts 'no' as her favourite word

Advanced skills
- Walks up stairs
- 'Helps' around the house
- Puts fingers to mouth and says 'shhh'

Toys and parental encouragement
If your child is already walking at this age you can encourage development of her motor skills by playing ball games – throwing and kicking it – and teaching her how to get down safely from things she has climbed on.

At 16 months
Mastered skills
- Turns the pages of a book
- Has temper tantrums when frustrated
- Becomes attached to a soft toy or other object

Emerging skills
- Stacks three bricks
- Discovers the joy of climbing
- Learns the correct way to use common objects (telephone etc)

Advanced skills
- Switches from two naps to one (if hasn't previously)
- Can take off a piece of clothing alone
- Gets fussy about food

Toys and parental encouragement
Continue to encourage all areas of development. The joy of temper tantrums will begin (if they haven't already). She will be testing your boundaries on anything and everything, from getting dressed and eating, to going to bed. As long as you are firm and consistent then small tantrums tend to remain that way and don't escalate into bigger ones, as she will understand her boundaries and the

behaviour you will and won't accept very quickly. The power of distraction is an amazing thing. Use it to your advantage when you sense a tantrum brewing!

At 17 months
Mastered skills
- Likes ride-on toys
- Enjoys pretend games
- Uses a handful of words regularly

Emerging skills
- Responds to directions, e.g., 'Sit down'
- Feeds doll
- Talks more clearly

Advanced skills
- Dances to music
- Sorts toys by colour, shape or size
- Kicks ball forward

Toys and parental encouragement
Continue to encourage her to follow simple instructions you give her. Even if she doesn't say many words herself at this stage, as long as you encourage her understanding then the speech should eventually follow. She will love imaginative play – feeding her doll or bear with a bottle, or spoon and pretend bowl of food, changing its nappy, etc.

At 18 months
Mastered skills
- Will 'read' board books alone
- Can pedal when put on a trike
- Scribbles well

Emerging skills
- Brushes teeth with help
- Strings words together in phrases
- Builds tower of four cubes

Advanced skills
- Throws ball overhead
- Takes toys apart then puts back together again
- Shows signs of toilet train readiness (aware of doing wee or poo in nappy)

Toys and parental encouragement
Encourage drawing as this will help her hand–eye coordination develop. If she is showing an awareness of going to the toilet in her nappy then you could buy a potty and have it in the bathroom upstairs, so she gets used to the sight of one. At bath time you can encourage her to sit on it if she wants to once you have taken her nappy off. Don't force her though – if she doesn't want to, that is fine. You could try encouraging her to put her teddy or dolly on the potty instead and talk about them doing a wee-wee or a poo-poo. All of this will sew the seed in her head as to what the potty will eventually be for.

At 19 months
Mastered skills
- Can run
- Can throw ball underarm
- Can use a spoon and fork well

Emerging skills
- Half of speech may be understandable
- Recognises when something is wrong (calling a dog a cat)

Advanced skills
- May know when she needs a wee
- Can wash and dry hands, and can brush teeth with help
- Can point to picture of dog or cat when you ask her to

Toys and parental encouragement
Continue with encouraging all areas of her development. Social-ising with other children at toddler groups and meeting up with friends who have children of similar ages is very helpful at this age. She will enjoy playing alongside and sometimes with other children, copying certain things they do. It will also be helpful to teach her to share, to prevent her becoming too selfish with toys.

At 20 months
Mastered skills
- Will pretend to feed a doll
- Can take off own clothes with help
- Will throw away an object such as rubbish, in imitation

Emerging skills
- Learns words at a rate of 10 or more per day
- Can walk up (but probably not down) stairs
- Searches for hidden objects

Advanced skills
- May start exploring genitals
- Draws straighter lines
- Can name several body parts

Toys and parental encouragement
Continue as above. Help to encourage her to practise removing and putting on her clothes, particularly trousers, in preparation for toilet training.

At 21 months
Mastered skills
- Can walk up stairs
- Enjoys helping around the house
- Can set simple goals, e.g., deciding to put a toy in a certain place

Emerging skills
- Can throw a ball overarm
- Can kick a ball
- Can make brick towers

Advanced skills
- Can name cat or dog when you show a picture
- Can make short sentences (me go ...)
- Can walk down stairs

Toys and parental encouragement
Most children at this age enjoy the bigger toys like ride-ons, things they can climb on, and toy kitchens and workbenches, where they can keep busy with the tools or pots and pans. Books and puzzles are also usually a big hit too once they have used up all of their energy.

At 22 months
Mastered skills
- Can kick a ball forward
- Follows two-step requests (get your doll and bring it here)
- Imitates others' behaviour

Emerging skills
- Can do simple puzzles
- Can draw a straight line
- Can identify several body parts

Advanced skills
- Can put on clothing
- Might be ready for a big bed
- Understands opposites (tall or short)

Toys and parental encouragement
Continue to encourage her to develop her independence – getting dressed, washing hands, brushing teeth – and moving to a big bed when she seems ready.

At 23 months
Mastered skills
- Can make a tower of four bricks
- Can name a simple picture in a book
- Can use 50 single words

Emerging skills
- Can sing simple tunes
- Takes more of an interest in playing with other children
- Can make two- or three-word sentences

Advanced skills
- Walks down stairs
- Asks 'why?'
- Talks about self (likes and dislikes)

Toys and parental encouragement
Continue to encourage sharing when playing with you and with other children. If you haven't already begun potty training then continue to encourage her to sit on the potty every now and then. Talk to her about what you are doing on the toilet every time you go (because inevitably you will have a 'shadow' watching you each time). Show her your wee or poo afterwards, and how you flush the toilet and wash your hands afterwards.

This will all teach her what happens ready for when you start toilet training her.

At 24 months
Mastered skills
- Can make short sentences
- Half of speech is understandable
- Can name at least six body parts on a doll

Emerging skills
- Can walk downstairs
- Starts talking about self
- Can arrange things in categories

Advanced skills
- Learns to jump
- Begins to understand concepts like 'soon' or 'later'
- Becomes attuned to gender differences

Toys and parental encouragement
Continue to encourage all areas of your child's development. Talk to her and give her lots of opportunities to listen and talk back. Provide activities where she can practise her physical skills too. She will be like a little sponge now, soaking up every bit of information you can give her and so eager to learn about the world and try most things physically – even if you think it may be beyond her. Encourage her with help or support if needed until she learns to be more independent at activities. Encourage her in everything through praise over the bits she gets right, rather than criticism over the parts she makes mistakes in.

The age at which your baby reaches the major physical milestones, like rolling, crawling, walking and even talking, can vary greatly. Below I have given a long-range time frame of when it is 'normal' for a baby to achieve one of the above milestones as long as she has no physical or mental disabilities or abnormalities.

Rolling: between 3 months and 12 months

Some very strong babies learn to roll from a very early age. However it is also perfectly normal for a baby to not actually roll completely over until much later. I had friends' babies who rolled over as young as three or four months but none of my three children rolled completely over until they were over seven months. They would happily kick their legs and roll from side to side, but were never interested in going any further. Don't be worried if your baby is the same.

Crawling: between 7 months and 13 months

Again, there is a very large time frame from when one particular baby may achieve this milestone to when another baby would – and both are completely normal. Some babies even miss this stage out altogether and either bum shuffle, commando crawl or go straight on to walking!

Walking: between 8 months and 18 months

Some babies will be off and walking from a very young age, others bide their time and take a lot longer. Once your baby learns to crawl or get around the room by some other means of movement, she will increase the speed at which she moves on a daily basis. Eventually she will get to the point where she can very easily get from one side of the room to the other in a matter of seconds. When this is the case, why would she waste her time practising something like walking, which is much slower and makes her feel very unstable on her feet? As long as she can bear her weight and doesn't seem to have any physical problems or difficulties with standing on her feet and walking along while holding on to your hands, then walking alone will come eventually when she feels brave enough, and is bored of having to crawl everywhere. I had one child walk at 11 months, one at 15 months, and one at 16 and a half months. They were, and are, all very 'normal' in terms of their physical development, and I wasn't worried at all, knowing they would begin walking when they were ready to.

Speech, vocalising and understanding

Speech is another area of development that varies greatly from child to child, and even among siblings. Sometimes if a child is excelling physically by crawling, walking and climbing from an early age then her speech may not be as advanced, as they are concentrating their efforts elsewhere. Even if your child doesn't say any recognisable words, as long as she is vocalising and babbling in her own little language, and can listen and follow simple verbal instructions that you give her, then she will begin saying new words when she is ready. Bilingual children who are being spoken to in more than one language at home (typically one language from the mother and a different one from the father), are renowned for developing vocabulary much later. If she can understand the speech you use and say to her and respond to it, then the actual language she uses herself will eventually come. Twins can develop language skills at a slower rate than single babies. You may also find that one twin talks and understands better than the other. This, again, is very normal and their sibling usually catches up, but if you are particularly worried then mention it to your health visitor.

It's so important to talk to your baby and toddler as much as possible. They learn by example, so she will vocalise much quicker if she is listening to your speech and can try to copy it. It's important you listen to her too, and give her opportunities to repeat simple words back to you as much as possible.

My first child and youngest were saying far more words than average by 18 months and could make their needs and wants very clearly known, using various words in their vocabulary. However my middle child was very different and, although he understood everything I said to him and could follow simple instructions, he barely said a word until he was over two years old! He then spent the next 12 months 'catching up' to where his brother and sister already were, and by the age of three was at the same point in his language development that his brother and other friends' children were, despite his late start.

In my opinion his late development was probably not helped by the fact that I didn't have as much time to spend teaching him words individually, like I had done with his older brother, as I had a very vocal toddler to deal with. Although Ollie heard language around him a lot, I didn't have a lot of time to spend with him on his own to give him as much opportunity to practise. When he was two years old his older brother went off to school so I was able to focus on Ollie 100 per cent and encourage his vocabulary. When I had my daughter, her brothers were both already at school full-time, so I have been able to spend a lot of time with her alone teaching and encouraging her speech, and I believe that is why she is able to express herself very well too.

9

Your questions answered

There are some questions that are always at the forefront of every mother's mind. I thought it would be a good idea to make a list of the most common questions I am asked, to make the answers easy for you to find.

Q: How much weight should my baby be gaining each week?
A: The average weight gain that babies commonly gain each week is between 6 and 8oz (175 and 225g) for the first few weeks. However some babies may only gain half of that amount weekly and others put on double. Both scenarios are perfectly normal. Most babies settle down a large weekly weight gain by around 8–10 weeks of age. All three of my breastfed babies gained almost one pound per week for the first 10 weeks. They then settled down to gaining between 4 and 6oz (115 and 175g) per week after that.

The centile charts that your baby's weight will be plotted on each time you take her to be weighed, to measure growth, are purely a guideline only. They were originally based on formula-fed babies, and have not been updated for a long time, so it's worth remembering this in particular if you are breastfeeding. Your baby will likely follow the same centile line that she was born on as you get her weighed regularly, but don't worry if she moves to the next one up or drops down to the one below. This can be due to growth spurts, illness or even burning off more calories as she starts to roll, crawl and walk around. As long as she's feeding regularly and gaining weight each week rather than losing it then you don't need to worry.

Q: How often should my baby poo per day?
A: Formula-fed babies tend to find a regular pattern of pooing very quickly – some may poo twice a day, others, one explosion every three days, and some, even once per week!

Breastfed babies can poo on average six to ten times per day for the first few weeks and it is normal for it to be a very watery yellow colour. Other breastfed babies may only poo once per day or even go a few days with no bowel movement. This is fine too – sometimes they don't poo as often because their body is just absorbing all of the nutrients contained in the breast milk they are drinking. (Although if your baby poos a lot it does not mean she isn't doing this too!) Ensure you are eating plenty of fruit and vegetables as this can have a major impact on your baby's bowel habits as well as your own when you are breastfeeding.

A baby's bowel habits can sometimes change when she gets to around six to eight weeks old. If she has been producing many soiled nappies on a daily basis this tends to settle down into a more regular pattern by this age. As long as she is producing plenty of wet nappies per day and doesn't seem uncomfortable in between periods of no soiled nappies then you don't need to be worried. When she does do a poo it should be easy to pass and soft, runny or loose – she is likely to make up for lost time if she does hold it in for a few days and give you a whole day of soiled nappies, so watch out!

Talk to your doctor if you are really worried about her not having a bowel movement for a longer period of time and if she seems uncomfortable with a swollen abdomen.

Q: My baby is taking 30 minutes on the first breast and 30 minutes on the second breast, but still seems hungry and just won't settle between feeds.

A: If she is taking the full amount of time on both breasts and still rooting around like she is hungry then the worry is that she is not getting an adequate amount of milk from the breast. Increase her time on the first breast to 45 minutes if you can to see if that helps. That should stimulate your breasts to produce more milk. If she is showing signs that the breast has been emptied (sucking, then pulling away and crying repeatedly), then your milk supply may not be enough to fill her up. You should be drinking a minimum of two litres of still water per day when breastfeeding and eating regular, well-balanced meals, containing items from all of the food groups. If you are doing or have tried all of the above then it might be worth offering your baby a small top-up of 1–2fl oz (30–60ml) after a breastfeed to see if she is still genuinely hungry. Ideally I would suggest you using expressed breast milk (EBM). If you managed to do some expressing in the early days when your milk was hopefully more plentiful then you could give that to her. If you don't have any EBM then you can offer your baby a formula top-up. Check with your health visitor as to which infant formula is currently recommended as being the closest to breast milk. If she takes 1–2fl oz (30–60ml) or more even after an hour or more of breastfeeding then it is likely that hunger was the cause. It may be that you only need to top-up with the bottle after the feeds later on in the day when your milk supply is lower. Introducing a permanent bottle of either EBM or formula at the 10:30 p.m. feed will also ensure she gets an adequate amount of milk to help her settle better at night-time. You should express fully and continue pumping until both breasts are empty at this time. See Chapter 4 for more details.

Q: At what age can I stop sterilising my baby's bottles?
A: The recommended guide is to continue sterilising bottles, breast pumps and feeding equipment until your baby is 12 months old. Sometimes, no matter how well you wash and clean them, milk deposits may be left behind in the teat of a bottle. Sterilising

ensures any germs are killed off to prevent your baby becoming more prone to illness while their immune system is still developing antibodies. However, most babies are crawling or even walking by 12 months so are regularly touching and exploring various places that may harbour germs. There is little point sterilising after this age so as long as any bottles or breast pumps and other feeding equipment are washed thoroughly with hot soapy water that is the best you can do.

Q: Do I need to sterilise my baby's weaning bowls and spoons?
A: Initially when you first begin weaning I would definitely advise that you sterilise all feeding equipment like the spoons and bowls your baby is directly eating from. Once she is crawling or aged over about eight months you can get away with just washing them thoroughly in hot soapy water. If you are too worried about not sterilising at all then you can pour boiling water into the bowl and rinse it out before placing food into it. You can also do the same with the spoon you plan to use, which will kill off any lurking germs.

Q: How long can breast milk be stored in the fridge or freezer before I need to use it?
A: It can be stored in the body of a fridge (not the door) for up to five days. You will then either need to use it or place in a sterilised breast milk freezer bag and place in the freezer until needed. Expressed breast milk can be stored in a combined fridge/freezer unit (with separate doors) for between three and six months at -18°C (-0.4°F). Please see Chapter 4 for more details on storing breast milk.

Q: How do I defrost breast milk?
A: There are two ways:
1: Get it out of the freezer the day before you need to use it and stand the bag or container with the EBM in upright in the fridge. By the following day it will have defrosted into liquid

form and you can pour it into a sterilised bottle ready to feed to your baby.

2: Stand the bag in a bowl of boiling water with a sterilised bottle ready next to it. As the iced milk melts, open the bag and transfer the liquid parts to the bottle immediately, pouring it into the bottle from the bag. Repeat this every time a little bit of the iced milk melts until the freezer bag is empty. It is important that you transfer the milk as soon as it melts, so that the liquid doesn't begin to heat up. If it does then you will have to throw it away, as baby milk shouldn't be reheated more than once. Place the cold defrosted EBM in the bottle in the body of the fridge until needed.

Q: At what age should I wean my baby on to solids? Is there a minimum age?

A: Current NHS and World Health Organization guidelines do not recommend parents begin solids until their baby is over 17 weeks, although they state that where possible you should encourage your baby to wait until six months. Weaning should only begin earlier than 17 weeks on the advice of your doctor or health visitor. Please see Chapter 6 for more information on signs that your baby may be ready.

Q: When can I give my baby cow's milk to drink?

A: Babies should not be given cow's milk to drink in a cup or bottle until they are over the age of 12 months. However it can be added to recipes that you are cooking for your baby; it is safe for her to have it in foods like cheese sauces, yoghurts, custard, etc., as long as she doesn't have a dairy intolerance.

Q: When can I move my baby from a rear-facing car seat to a forward-facing one?

A: It really depends on the type of rear-facing seat you have and which 'stage' it comes under in the retailer's guide. A group 0 seat is for babies up to 10kg (22lb), which is roughly from birth to six to nine months. A group 0+ is for babies up to 13kg (29lb), roughly from birth to 12–18 months. They can both be used in the front or rear of the car, but it is safer to put them in the rear. It is illegal to carry a child in a rear-facing child seat in the front if the vehicle is protected by an active passenger airbag. Rear-facing seats provide greater protection for the baby's head, neck and spine than forward-facing seats, so it is best to keep your baby in one of these for as long as possible. Only move them to a forward-facing one once they have exceeded the maximum weight for the baby seat or the top of their head is higher than the top of the seat. The law requires all children travelling in cars to use the correct child restraint until either 135cm (4ft 5in) in height or 12 years (whichever is sooner). The seat must meet the United Nations Standard ECE 44-03.

Q: At what age should I move my baby from the Moses basket to the cot?

A: There is no right or wrong age, or a particular time to do it that will be the same for every baby. Certain factors may affect how quickly the decision is made: her disturbing you with her baby noises as she sleeps, or even you and your partner disturbing her. A big factor for some parents that forces them to make the decision is how quickly the baby gains weight and outgrows it. My eldest had to be moved to the big cot at six weeks as he completely filled the basket and could barely move around in it any more, whereas my middle child stayed in it until 10 weeks, and my youngest moved to the big cot when she was eight weeks old. When you do move her into the big cot you may need to put some rolled-up towels in there on either side of her to make her cosier, as it will feel very big in comparison to her Moses basket and she may be unsettled if you don't. Trial her during her day sleeps at the beginning without any rolled-up towels. If she sleeps happily in the cot like that then progress to putting her to sleep in the big cot for her 7–10 p.m. evening sleep. After three nights of still settling and sleeping well for all of her day sleeps and evening sleep then you can begin also using the cot for her to sleep in between 11 p.m. and 7 a.m., and there will be no need to use the Moses basket again. If you do need to use the rolled-up towels to begin with as you make the transition from Moses basket to cot, you need to gradually take them out as she begins to move around the cot more and more. Again, do it over a period of days and start by removing during the day sleeps first, then progress to the evening and finally core night sleep.

Q: When is a good time and age to move my baby into the nursery rather than in the same room as me?
A: The current recommendation by The Lullaby Trust and the NHS is to keep your baby sleeping in the same room as you for the first six months. I have found this is again a very personal decision. I've known some parents to do this after a week or two, as their baby is such a noisy sleeper that they hardly manage to sleep at all while sharing a room. Equally I've known others who are still sharing a room when their baby is six months. My recommendation is to coincide this move to the nursery with the transition from Moses basket to the big cot – so somewhere between 6 and 12 weeks. If you do the transition while your baby is still under 12 weeks then you shouldn't have any issues with her being unsettled by 'the move!'

Q: How long should I breastfeed for?
A: The Department of Health recommendations are as follows:

- Mothers should breastfeed exclusively for the first six months.
- Six months is also the recommended age for the introduction of solids for both breastfed and formula-fed infants.
- Mothers who are unable to, or choose not to follow these recommendations, should be supported to optimise their infant's nutrition.

- Breastfeeding (and/or breast milk substitutes if used) should continue beyond the first six months along with appropriate types and amounts of solid food.

The above are recommendations. However, when and how you stop breastfeeding may be influenced by many factors: milk supply, lifestyle, lack of weight gain, returning to work, etc. It will be an entirely individual choice for each mother and baby. You will know when the time is right to stop for whatever reason. Even if you don't manage to meet the recommended guidelines, every day and week that you have breastfed your baby will have given her immune system a boost with the extra antibodies and nutrition you have provided her with over that period of time.

Q: How many ounces of milk per day should my baby be drinking?
A: If your baby is under 12 months then the recommended daily milk intake is a minimum of 20fl oz (600ml) but between 20 and 25fl oz (600–700ml). Once you introduce solids this daily allowance can be made up of the breast milk or infant formula that your baby drinks, as well as the milk used in any foods you give her to eat, like cheese sauces, yoghurts and custard, among other things.

Once she is over 12 months the recommended daily milk intake drops to 10–12fl oz (300–360ml) per day, which is roughly one or two cups of milk.

Q: How do I know if my baby has a temperature? What should her normal body temperature be?
A: A normal body temperature for a baby or child can be from 35–37.5°C (95–99.5°F). The favoured temperature to aim for is 37°C (98.6°F) so if her temperature has dropped to 35°C (95°F) then you may want to consider putting an extra layer of clothing on her to warm her up. Always take her temperature twice to ensure the accuracy of the reading. An underarm digital thermometer

or a digital ear thermometer are the best ones to use for children (see page 21), as they are less intrusive and give a fast reading, although the digital ear thermometer is not recommended to be used on babies under six months as it is difficult to obtain an accurate reading. Any reading over 38°C (100.4°F) is considered a temperature. If your baby's temperature is only slightly over 38°C (100.4°F) then you could try removing some of her clothing and then re-check her temperature 10 minutes later to see if it has come down. If it hasn't and she seems unwell and showing other symptoms then contact your doctor for advice on what to do next.

Q: Can I drink alcohol while breastfeeding? How much is safe?
A: Levels of alcohol in breast milk remain close to those in the mother's bloodstream. Levels will be at their highest between 30 and 60 minutes after drinking, or 90 minutes if you have been drinking with a meal. It takes two to three hours for a unit of alcohol (small glass of wine or half a pint of ordinary-strength beer) to leave a nursing mum's milk. While large amounts of alcohol in breast milk can have a sedative effect, it is more likely to make your baby agitated and disrupt sleep patterns. Alcohol inhibits a mother's let down (the release of milk from the nipple). Studies have shown that babies take around 20 per cent less milk if there is alcohol present, so they'll need to feed more often, although some have been known to go on a 'nursing strike', probably because of the altered taste of the milk.

Dr Wendy Jones, a pharmacist who is a registered breastfeeding supporter with the UK-based Breastfeeding Network says it's safe for breastfeeding mothers to drink alcohol 'within reason' – a position supported by La Leche League and the American Academy of Pediatrics' Committee on Drugs. She says, 'an occasional glass of wine is fine but binge or regular drinking above the daily unit guidelines of two to three alcohol units is harmful to Mum and Baby. It is better not to drink every day but keep alcohol for social occasions.' If you do overdo it on one of these social occasions then breastfeeding probably isn't wise. 'If you feel drunk, and particularly if you have drunk enough to vomit, it is better not to breastfeed for a long enough period of time to allow the alcohol to leave your milk', Wendy advises. Alcohol is not locked into breast milk so 'pumping and dumping' (expressing and discarding milk) is unnecessary. 'The mum may need to express milk off for comfort, but as the alcohol level in her own body falls, the level will also fall in her milk. Breast milk from a mother who has the occasional small glass of wine or half a pint of beer is still superior to formula milk, which does not contain all the immunological and other special properties we know breast milk has.'

Q: I have one breast bigger than the other, which seems to produce more milk. How do I increase milk supply on the smaller breast? Should I put my baby to that breast more often than the other?
A: You should always aim to feed evenly off each breast, as discussed in Chapter 4 (see page 74). To increase supply in the smaller breast you can try expressing 1fl oz (30ml) off that breast BEFORE a feed and then put your baby straight on to that breast. By pumping before feeding you are encouraging your breast to make more milk as your baby will stimulate the breast at the end of the feed. If you tried pumping *after* a feed it is very unlikely you will be unable to express anything off as your baby will have emptied it. This is because a baby's suck at the breast is much more effective and likely to increase supply. Offer the expressed milk to her from a bottle after the feed, if she still seems hungry, in the first few days that you begin this increased milk plan, as it will take that long for your breasts to catch up with the increase in demand. Once you begin to make a bit more milk then you may be able to freeze this excess expressed milk that your baby doesn't need to drink.

Q: My baby prefers one breast over the other and is always fussing when feeding from the opposite one. What do I do?
A: Every baby I have worked with, including my own three children, seems to show a preference for one breast over the other.

It generally tends to be your better producing one too. Even though they show a clear preference it is very important that you feed evenly off each breast by swapping her over at each feed and starting from the opposite breast that you did at the feed previously. You can try various positions to encourage her to feed better from the breast she prefers less. The rugby ball hold can sometimes trick her into thinking that she is still feeding from her preferred breast – for a little while at least. Unfortunately it is something that you just have to persevere with and know that she is going to be a bit more difficult to feed on one side in particular. You are not alone though and it is perfectly normal for her to show a preference.

Q: I'm breastfeeding and always worrying about how much my baby is drinking and if it is enough? How do I know that I am satisfying her?
A: This is every breastfeeding mother's biggest worry and one that we can all relate to. As long as your baby seems satisfied between feeds after being offered a full feed using both breasts as described in Chapter 4, happily waits three to four hours until the next feed and is sleeping fairly well at night, then she is taking enough. It is a good idea to get her weighed weekly or fortnightly during the first month or so to ensure that she is also putting on weight. It varies from baby to baby in how much weight they put on regularly, but the crucial thing is not how much weight she puts on, but that she is putting on weight rather than losing it. As long as she is doing this then you can be sure she is satisfied – she would soon let you know if she wasn't.

If she doesn't seem settled and is still rooting around quite soon after a feed, then I would suggest you try to encourage her to spend longer on the first breast, to ensure she gets more of the important hind milk to fill her up. This will help her to feel more satisfied.

Q: At what age can I expect my baby to drop her night feed, and start sleeping for longer periods at night-time?
A: I think this must be one of the top questions on every parent's list! The answer to this will depend on your routine on a daily

basis, how well she is feeding and how quickly you establish good sleeping habits and associations to enable her to sleep for longer periods of time. Potentially, if you get all of these things right and establish a good feeding and sleep routine as early as possible, then your baby could be ready to drop her night feed around the age of 10 weeks. Refer to Chapters 4 and 5 for more information on how to establish a good feeding and sleep routine, and details on how to drop the night feed effectively.

Q: My baby seems full of wind and uncomfortable most of the time. What can I do to help her?
A: First of all it is important to ensure that you are not snack feeding her and giving her small feeds too frequently. This will make her more prone to pain from wind, as each feed will not have long enough for her tummy to digest and the air bubbles to settle, before more milk is added. See the Chapter 4 for more information on how to structure her feeds.

Products like gripe water, Infacol and Dentinox can help with breaking down the trapped air bubbles and preventing wind pain if your baby is uncomfortable and struggles to burp.

If you are breastfeeding then you need to be aware that certain foods you eat can affect your baby's digestive system massively. Chapter 4 also has more details on foods to avoid that can trigger excess wind problems.

Q: My newborn baby will not go down in the Moses basket for any length of time and just cries unless we hold her or she is moving in the car or pushchair. She calms down and is happy as soon as my husband or I hold her though ...
A: This is very normal when your baby is newborn. She has been used to being snuggled and cosy inside your womb, surrounded by lots of reassuring noises and sounds, both from your body and the outside world. To be expected to make the jump from that, to just being put down to sleep in a Moses basket or cot, in a quiet

dark room on her own as soon as she is born is just too much of a change. Using the method of placing rolled-up towels in her Moses basket and wedging her in between those will make her feel cuddled, and she will be less likely to startle awake. White noise will also be a reassuring and familiar noise for her to hear. The pat-and-shhh technique will also encourage her to get used to sleeping in the basket happily too. At times only a reassuring cuddle from you will do though, and it is important that you indulge her with this. This will help her to feel loved and comforted and she will gain more confidence in sleeping alone if she knows you will cuddle her when she needs it. All of this is described in more detail in Chapter 5.

Q: When is the best time to introduce a bottle to my breastfed baby? My midwife advised me not to at all as it will put my baby off the breast.

A: Many people advise mothers not to give their baby a bottle at all, as they say it is likely to put them off wanting to breastfeed. This is completely wrong information and totally untrue. It is important to get your baby established on the breast and feeding well at regular intervals. Once this has been achieved, usually between 7 and 14 days after birth, then your baby can be offered a bottle at any time after that, and there will be no risk at all that she will go off breastfeeding, as long as you continue to have a good supply for her. I, along with every mother I have worked for, have given our babies a regular daily bottle from the age of two weeks at the latest. Not one of those babies has shown a preference for the bottle over the breast and gone off breastfeeding. This is based on hundreds of babies! The higher risk is that if you don't introduce a regular bottle, she will get to the stage where she will refuse a bottle at all. It's important to introduce a bottle by the age of four weeks at the latest to prevent any reluctance from her towards taking it. More information on this can be found in Chapter 4 (see page 122).

Q: Does controlled crying affect my baby emotionally in any way?

A: The short answer to this question is no – not if the technique is used correctly. A baby needs to know that you will respond to her needs. There is, however, a big difference between responding to her 'needs' and giving in to her 'wants'. As a parent you will quickly learn to recognise when your baby is very upset, and when she is just crying because she is tired. Leaving her to self-soothe and try to settle herself as she gets older will benefit her ability to sleep much better, long term. I would never advise any parent to attempt controlled crying on a baby under six weeks though – they are too young, and it rarely works because they don't understand what you are doing. More details on how to establish good sleep associations and the controlled-crying and timed comforting methods can be found in Chapter 5.

Q: What is the most effective way to treat teething pain?

A: There are many teething products that can be bought from various places all claiming to be the best at treating teething pain. I have tried many of them and the one that I have found most effective is the Anbesol teething liquid (not the gel form). It can be bought from most pharmacies, online or in some supermarkets. With it being a liquid it can be applied directly to the gums, and it doesn't slide off as teething gel tends to. I have found this works 90 per cent of the time, but infant paracetamol and Nurofen are also good to have in the house to use when the pain is very bad.

Q: Is it okay to feed a formula bottle at night instead of breastfeeding so that my partner can do it and allow me some sleep?

A: If your baby is breastfed and only having expressed breast milk during the daytime then I would advise against giving a bottle of formula in the middle of the night. Formula can sometimes sit heavier on a baby's tummy and make them feel fuller for a longer period. The night feed is the first feed most parents want to drop, so it is not a good idea to make her feel very full at that time or it will be more difficult to reduce that feed and then drop it. If you would like to introduce a bottle of formula then the best time to do it would be at the 10–11 p.m. feed. This will be the best time to try to fill her up as much as possible in the hope that she will sleep well into the night, before needing another feed. If you express your breast milk off at this time, while your partner feeds your baby a bottle of formula, then the expressed breast milk can either be placed in a bottle and used for the middle-of-the-night feed, or stored and used at a later date. Where possible always try to stick to expressed breast milk in a bottle for the night feed.

Q: My baby cries a lot in the evenings, and nothing seems to soothe her until she eventually passes out. My doctor has diagnosed colic. We are very stressed as we never seem to get an evening any more that isn't filled with an upset screaming baby. What can we do to change things?
A: The first thing I would suggest is that you read Chapter 4, and if your baby isn't already established on a regular feeding routine, then you need to try to steer her towards that. Snack feeding can cause a lot of colic pain in babies so it is vital that babies are encouraged towards taking full feeds every three to four hours to give their tummy time to digest their milk and the air bubbles to settle. Once you have established a good feeding routine then you need to also ensure that she is sleeping well during the day in a quiet, dark environment. If a baby has only cat-napped all day then by the evening she can become so overtired that she will just cry inconsolably. An overtired baby will behave in a very similar way to a baby genuinely suffering from colic. Many parents who have contacted me regarding babies who have been diagnosed with colic due to excessive crying find that as soon as they establish a good feeding and sleep routine their baby's temperament completely changes, and the 'colic' disappears.

If your baby is already following the sleep and feeding routine discussed in those chapters then it may be worth looking towards possible allergies or intolerances that could be causing the pain and crying. If you are breastfeeding then you should look carefully at your diet. There are many foods that can trigger reactions in your baby. If you are bottle-feeding then it may be that your baby has lactose or cow's milk intolerance. More details can be found in Chapter 4 about all of this (see page 110).

Q: I always put my baby down to sleep on her side or back, but every time I go in to check on her she has rolled on to her tummy and is fast asleep. Should I roll her back again?

A: Once your baby has learned to roll over, it is perfectly safe to allow her to sleep on her tummy if that is her preferred position. If she can roll, then she also must be old enough to hold her head up well and turn her head to the side in a purposeful movement. You can put her down to sleep on her side or back if that helps relieve your anxiety, but she will always roll to a position she finds most comfortable in her sleep, or to settle herself to sleep. Rolling her over on to her back or side when you check on her is fine to do if you want to, but you do risk unsettling and waking her up. If you haven't already introduced a sleeping bag or grobag for sleep times and have been using blankets to cover your baby at night, then you may want to reconsider. Once a baby is rolling and moving around in the cot then it is safer to take any blankets away and just use a sleeping bag to keep her temperature regulated at sleep and naptimes.

Q: My baby is 16 weeks. She has dropped her night feed about three weeks ago but has started waking around 5 a.m. and is very unsettled. She does resettle if I cuddle her back to sleep. Should I just leave her to cry?

A: All babies and children come into a light sleep from 5 a.m. until they finally wake fully around 7 a.m. There are various factors that could disturb her while she is in this light sleep and cause her to wake fully. At 16 weeks she is getting close to an age when you could potentially begin weaning. If she has just begun waking at 5 a.m. it could be due to her beginning to get a little bit hungry. Babies do have another growth spurt at 16 weeks. However, the quick cuddle in bed with you helps to just push her through that extra couple of hours. You could try increasing her day feeds by putting an extra ounce in each bottle-feed or encouraging her to spend longer on the breast at each feed. If her 10–11 p.m. feed is being given as a bottle-feed then also increasing the amount she has at this time should also help. If it has been hunger that wakes her then increasing her feeds will solve the early-morning waking. Other things that can cause early-morning waking are being too cold, having a soiled nappy that has leaked on to her clothes or teething. Please see Chapter 5 (page 220) for further information on how to solve these problems.

Q: My baby can regularly be heard at 4–5 a.m. chatting away over the monitor. She doesn't cry and eventually just goes back to sleep. Should I go to her or just leave her?
A: If she is happy to chat for a little while in the night and then go back to sleep then you don't need to go in to her. If she begins to cry after chatting for a while, then it may be that there is a problem and you need to go in and do your usual checks of her nappy, position in the bed, if she has her comfort blanket or toy, wind, etc. Once you are satisfied that she is okay, then repeat your usual settling process and walk out of the room.

Q: My baby is five months and has just begun to get a bit fussy when taking the bottle. She will drink the first few ounces but then when I stop to wind her she doesn't seem that bothered about drinking any more, and cries and gets upset if I try to persevere.
A: It may be that you need to increase the teat size that you are using. All bottles have teats that vary in the flow and speed that the milk comes out of the teat. As your baby gets older and more efficient at feeding then you need to increase the flow of milk by

moving her to the next sized teat. The biggest indicator of when this needs to happen is that she will become fussy and almost bored of drinking her milk once her initial hunger is satisfied. This is described in more detail in Chapter 4 (see page 96). Alternatively, if increasing her teat size doesn't encourage her to take any extra milk then she may just be happy taking a smaller amount. As long as she continues to put weight on, and you always encourage her to wait a fair amount of time between feeds rather than resort to snack feeding her, then you don't need to worry. Babies will never starve themselves – they eat when they are hungry. If she doesn't want to finish her feed, but is still happy to wait a few hours before having her next one, then she is obviously taking enough to satisfy her current growth needs.

Q: My baby is six months and still fully swaddled. If I try to put him down unswaddled he wakes frequently as he doesn't like it. Surely he can't sleep swaddled forever? Any suggestions?
A: I have known some parents to still be swaddling their baby at eight or nine months old. It is likely that the older he gets and begins to move around the cot, then he will naturally escape from the swaddle anyway, and learn to sleep happily without it. If you would like to try an alternative to swaddling then you could buy a grobag with long arms. These are perfect for babies who like the security of a swaddle, and become unsettled when allowed their arms free. If you buy a slightly bigger size, then the arms of the grobag tend to be so long that they cover your baby's hands. As it is having their hands free that tends to unsettle them, the problem is solved. As with all sleep changes, always trial the grobag for day sleeps first, progressing to the evening sleep and then the full night-time sleep, as your baby becomes happy and used to it. See Chapter 5 for more information.

Q: I'm having night-time nappy trouble. My little boy, who is 13 months, keeps waking up soaked through – his clothes and sheet are thoroughly wet. I have tried changing nappy size

but it got worse, so now I have gone back to the original size I was using. I use Pampers and I always put a fresh nappy on him just before putting him in his cot at 7 p.m.

A: I have always put two nappies on my babies once they started sleeping for 12 hours a night. I encountered this exact same problem with my firstborn 10 years ago. Like you, I tried various solutions but in the end I put two nappies on him and it worked – we never had a leaky nappy after that. You can put one nappy on top of the other. You don't actually use any extra nappies as the one on top can be put on your baby in the morning if clean. It will still be dry 90 per cent of the time – it is just there as a safety net.

Q: Do babies tend to be less keen on drinking milk the older they get? My little one is over 10 months and is really starting to cut down on his milk intake. He is still taking plenty of solids and I am including more milk in cooking so he doesn't cut back too much. Should I be worried?

A: Some babies are real milk monsters and others the opposite and begin to reduce the amount of milk that they want to drink on their own. As long as he is getting the minimum amount recommended for his age, which is around 20fl oz (600ml) a day for a baby under one year, then I wouldn't worry. When he is over one year, the minimum amount drops to 10–12fl oz (300–360ml) or two cups of milk. You can also then change him over to full-fat cow's milk to drink. Some babies prefer this and pick up on their milk intake again. I wouldn't worry if he is a healthy weight and getting plenty of milk via the meals he is eating anyway.

Q: At times I am finding it really difficult to settle my baby after a feed. He is four weeks old and I breastfeed him for all of his feeds apart from the 10:30 p.m., when we give him a bottle of EBM. He feeds very well, but won't always settle with me. Even after a full breastfeed he is rooting around on me, but as soon as I offer him the breast he refuses and doesn't seem hungry. When I hand him to my husband, he is

usually able to settle him fairly quickly. As his mother I am finding it very frustrating that he won't always settle with me and don't understand why. Help!

A: This a very common occurrence for breastfeeding mothers to experience. The smell of your breast milk is very strong to your baby only. It can drive him positively wild if he knows you are nearby and you are trying to stall him for a feed. A bit like waving a carrot in front of a donkey but not allowing them to have it! Even after a feed, a baby can still be unsettled by that enticing smell when being cuddled by the mother. They don't actually want any more milk but the scent of having it nearby is all a bit confusing and can make it difficult for them to relax enough to fall asleep. Most of the time, your comforting milk smell will be something they enjoy.

If you find yourself in the type of scenario described above, then handing your baby to your partner is the best option. They will certainly enjoy the extra time they get to bond with your little one and it will give them and you confidence to know that your baby can be settled by someone other than you.

Having breastfed all three of my babies I understand exactly what you are describing all too well. There were times that I would go in to do the night feed with my little one and we would be all done very quickly. However, the amount of time I would need to spend trying to settle my baby would feel like it took forever at times. I didn't want to have to wake my husband who needed some sleep at least before going off to work in the morning, but there were times when I had to as our baby just wouldn't settle on me. The times that I did hand over the rein, our little one would be asleep on his chest within minutes, leaving me feeling frustrated that I had been trying to achieve just that for the previous hour! Every breastfeeding mother that I have worked with has also experienced this scenario at times. It generally only lasts for the first three to four months of breastfeeding, when your baby is very young, and isn't a permanent thing.

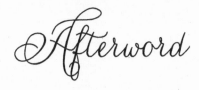

Afterword

I hope you all enjoyed reading my book and found the information informative and helpful. My aim in writing *The Blissful Baby Expert* was to provide parents with one book that they could use for reference when needing answers to all the important everyday things that crop up when looking after a small baby. All of the tips and experiences that I have had and learned, both professionally while caring for other people's babies and personally with my own children, are contained in this book. This advice will help to ensure that those first precious weeks and months with your new baby are as relaxed and as enjoyable as they can possibly be.

I am always happy to advise further and more specifically and can be contacted through my website – www.theblissfulbabyexpert. co.uk – Twitter or my Facebook page.

Wishing you all 'blissful babies' and the best of luck.

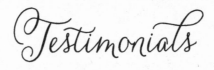

Testimonials

Below is just a small selection of the feedback comments and testimonials that parents have written about me after I have finished working with them and their baby:

Lisa worked for us as a night maternity nurse for my daughter Tabitha. Based on my experience I cannot recommend her highly enough. Endlessly patient and wonderfully practical, Lisa has a genuine love of small babies. However, while affectionate and loving with our daughter, she is sympathetic to the role of mum, and never made me feel anything other than the most important person in Tabitha's life. Lisa is there to support and help not take over (unless you want or need her to). I have heard it said by so many new parents, 'Where is the instruction manual?' Well, here it is: Lisa. She has an amazing understanding of the way small babies work, while remaining ever attentive and alive to the needs of each individual baby. At 10 weeks Tabitha is a happy, smiling and content little baby – and that is all thanks to Lisa. Lisa is so much more than just a maternity nurse and she does so much more than just work nights. Not only does Lisa teach you how to care for your child, she is also a fantastic support for the parents, in particular for Mum. Regularly responding to panic-stricken text messages in the middle of the night, Lisa has always been there on the end of the phone to help get us through, particularly in those first few weeks when it is all so new. She has been a lifeline and a true friend and I am confident that she will be a welcome and valued addition to any family. We will miss her.

Kate, mother to Tabitha

In all honesty, I do not think that we could have survived the first three months without Lisa. Not only was she fantastic with our daughter Orla, she was fantastic with both my husband and me. As a first-time mum, handling a newborn was extremely daunting and quite overwhelming. Lisa was there 24 hours a day if we needed her and was always ready to offer guidance and support, as well as giving us some much-needed sleep! Lisa was confident in her approach and set clear guidelines for establishing a routine early on. If things went wrong – as they often did – she was flexible and calm and soon got us back on track again. Lisa combined her training and experience as a nanny with a real empathy gained from having young children of her own. She understood the dilemmas a new mum feels and was sympathetic to the changing patterns of young babies (they don't often do what the books say!). She was also confident with Orla; they had a great relationship, which gave me confidence too. I learnt a lot from her

Jane, Mother to Orla

Lisa is a gentle and caring person and our boys seemed very happy with her and settled down fairly quickly when she was around. Lisa introduced a feeding and sleeping routine to the boys, which encouraged them to sleep better at night. Both parents were able to sleep through the night knowing that their children were in safe, capable hands. She was also very adept at feeding and managing both boys simultaneously!

Tina, mother to twin boys Daniel and Michael

Lisa's knowledge and experience has been invaluable in getting the girls to sleep for longer at night and developing our routines as they grow. She is on the end of the phone with advice even when she is not working for us. The girls respond very well to her firm but hugely caring manner.

Debra, mother to twin girls Charlotte and Anya

As a first-time mum I found Lisa's support and advice invaluable in order to adjust to motherhood. Lisa started working with us when Jacob was two weeks old and immediately we became more settled as a family and not just because we got a decent night's sleep. She was very professional and reliable in her duties, and helped establish a routine that made coping with those early weeks so much easier for us all, particularly when it came to breastfeeding a very hungry boy who liked to snack and doze!

Emma, mother to Jacob

Lisa has been a wonderful support to us since the arrival of our son Harry. She has offered sound advice and made the early months of having a newborn baby a lot less stressful as a result. In particular, having Lisa a couple of nights a week has enabled me to maintain my energy levels for our two older children. Most importantly for me, with her help and advice I have successfully breastfed Harry, which is something I struggled with, with our other two children.

Claire, mother to Harry

Lisa started when Max was about five weeks old and was waking up two, maybe more, times at night. I was very keen to establish Max on a good sleeping and eating routine and get him to sleep through the night as early as possible. Lisa immediately made me feel like I was in the hands of an expert. She was able to settle Max quickly and quietly and gave me very helpful suggestions concerning all aspects of Max's development. I was very impressed by the fact that I never heard Max cry, even when I slept in the room next door, so I was able to get some much-needed sleep. Having two nights of unbroken sleep totally transformed my days with Max as my life returned to normal. Lisa would always get in touch the day after she stayed with us to explain how she looked after him and to give useful tips – e.g., put Max to sleep on his side or keep him awake properly at the 10.30 p.m. feed.

Vicky, mother to Max

Lisa came to work for us as a maternity nurse six weeks after our son, Joseph, was born. At the time we employed Lisa, we thought she would simply provide night nurse cover and allow us to get some sleep. However, not only did Lisa do this, but she also provided a great deal more – she devised a fantastic and practical routine for us to follow, covering feeding, sleeping and playing, which Joseph took to so well that within eight weeks we had our evenings back and by 10 weeks he was sleeping through. Lisa also provided us with advice by email, text and phone whenever we needed it, which, as first-time parents, has been invaluable. Lisa's wealth of experience with babies means that she can deal with any issue which comes up and provide a practical solution. Lisa is punctual, totally trustworthy and fun to have around.

I suffered from post-natal depression and Lisa helped me to overcome it by offering advice, support and kindness and always making herself available to discuss problems. She went above and beyond to help me and put me in touch with people who had experienced PND themselves. We cannot recommend her highly enough.

Antonia, mother to Joe

Lisa was of enormous help from the start. Before Hugo was born, she had already sent a feeding schedule to help out.

The first night Lisa came, she helped me rearrange his Moses basket and helped with his feeding schedule and taught me how to swaddle him properly, which improved his sleeping a lot.

I got help on how to get him to sleep through the night as well as helping me with his daytime naps. Lisa also advised on his feeding and when to start weaning him.

Whenever I had a question or problem I could email her and I always got a prompt and reassuring response to any of my queries. Lisa also always enquired after Hugo to see how he was doing whenever we had made a change to his sleeping or feeding schedule or when he had not been himself.

She has taught me how to deal with Hugo in every aspect.

Due to her Hugo has become a contented boy, who sleeps and eats well and is very happy and sociable.

Lisa also took care of him for four nights, so my husband and I could spend some time together. She always updated me on his progress and Hugo seemed very happy to be there with her and her family.

Celine, mother to Hugo

Lisa was a joy and her calm and competent nature has made our first months such a happy and special time. She has helped and guided us with all aspects of baby care, from feeding and sleep routines for day and night, sterilising, bottle-feeding, expressing, settling baby, etc. She basically looked after Imogen during the nights, getting her into a routine and giving me a wonderful night's sleep. During the day she acted as a sort of baby consultant, guiding us and resolving any problems that arose in her absence. Lisa has a natural gift with babies and was invaluable. She was highly reliable, prompt and fun to have around. I cannot recommend Lisa highly enough.

Rebecca, mother to Imogen

References

NHS Direct website
www.nhsdirect.nhs.uk

BabyCentre website
www.babycentre.co.uk

Mumsnet website
www.mumsnet.com

Drinkaware website
www.drinkaware.co.uk

Kate Kripke article. May
2012, 'The difference
between Normal Postpartum
adjustment and PPD'
www.postpartumprogress.com

The Lullaby Trust website
www.lullabytrust.org.uk

Murdoch Childrens Research
Institute
www.mcri.edu.au

Helpful websites where you
can buy equipment
www.mothercare.com
www.amazon.co.uk
www.toysrus.co.uk (and then
click on the Babies R Us
section)

Angelcare movement and
sound monitor
http://angelcarebaby.com

Avent bottles and breast
pumps
www.avent.philips.com

Tommee Tippee first cups
www.tommeetippee.co.uk

Annabel Karmel recipes
www.annabelkarmel.com

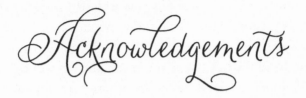

Acknowledgements

First of all I would like to thank all of the wonderful parents and babies who I have been so privileged to work with and look after. Each one, with their individuality, has taught me something new, and seeing how happy and thriving they are on a daily basis once it is time to move on to a new family makes all of our patience and perseverance so worthwhile.

Special thanks go to Sally and Toby Davis, parents to twin boys Miles and Samuel. I began working for them just as I began writing my book. With their constant encouragement and support when the end seemed so far away, I was always motivated to keep going. They deserve complete credit for the original book cover design when the idea of the book was only just beginning – I can't thank them enough and really appreciate all of their input in helping me and my editor achieve the finished product.

Many thanks also to Cherry Reynard, another of the parents I worked for, who is mother to Hannah and Lexi. Her editing input was a huge help in structuring the information I wanted to give in a clear, concise way, without my usual long-winded, round the houses descriptions. She also wrote the lovely foreword, which is very much appreciated.

I would also like to thank Gaz Roberts for the fantastic illustrations he did. The original illustrations have been re-drawn by my publishers but Gaz gave us a starting point to work from. He matched my descriptions in picture form perfectly and I am very grateful he found the time to help me out, despite being very busy caring for his own twins and having various work projects demanding deadlines from him.

Thanks also to my editor Susanna Abbott for taking the time to read the manuscript, seeing the potential of the valuable information I was giving, and believing in me and my book: I thank her from the bottom of my heart. She has worked with me every step of the way and helped me to improve the way I deliver the information in *The Blissful Baby Expert.* She has answered all of my annoying questions along the way, as her assistant Catherine Knight, and they have both supported me and the decisions I've made about the book. Thank you so much for making my dream of having my book published a reality!

My final thanks and appreciation go to my ever-loving husband, Martin. He has always supported my work completely and understood how involved I need to be as I regularly respond to panic-stricken messages and calls at all hours of the day and night. He has even become involved himself when I have literally bought my work home with me – we have had many of the babies I work with, including sets of twins, come and stay with us in our family home while their parents were away or ill. He is amazing and I wouldn't be the person I am today without him by my side.

Not forgetting of course our three gorgeous children: Jack, Ollie and Loren. They have taught me the most and are all very individual and different in their own way. In having the experience with my own babies to draw on, I am certain that this has made the vital difference to how understanding and empathetic I am towards the mothers and babies that I work with.

I hope one day my children will all read this book and be as proud of me as I am of them all each and every day while watching them grow. Mummy loves you all to the moon and back.

XXX

Index